# Patient Safety and Serious Incident Responses

This step-by-step guide takes the reader through the complex process of investigating serious incidents in health, social care, and criminal justice environments, acknowledging differences of culture and context that shape an investigation. Taking a multi-disciplinary approach, Part 1 begins by exploring the key principles of investigation, including ethical and legal perspectives, the involvement of families and carers, and being aware of unconscious bias, amongst other issues. Part 2 outlines in detail the conduct of investigations, from planning to processing the findings, before moving on to Part 3, carrying them out in diverse settings.

Further chapters then look at investigating within diverse environments before moving on to Part 4 which deals with reviewing and analysing the evidence collected and writing up the investigation. This final part also examines the pivotal issue of learning from the investigation and disseminating the report. The inclusion of case studies, models of good practice, and vignettes enables the reader to view each stage of the process in context and drive the transformation of practice.

This practical resource is designed to support health and social care professionals who undertake investigations as part of their role, including nurses, allied health practitioners, social workers, doctors, and psychologists, as well as military personnel and law enforcers. It is an essential companion.

**Alison Elliott** is a Senior Lecturer at the University of Central Lancashire and Programme Lead: Offender Personality Disorder Programme.

**Karen M. Wright** is Professor Emerita at the University of Central Lancashire, practicing psychotherapist, Chair of an NHS research Ethics Committee, and registered nurse.

# Patient Safety and Serious Incident Responses

The Essentials

**Edited by**
**Alison Elliott and Karen M. Wright**

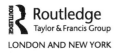

Routledge
Taylor & Francis Group

LONDON AND NEW YORK

Cover design: © Getty

First published 2025
by Routledge
4 Park Square, Milton Park, Abingdon, Oxon OX14 4RN

and by Routledge
605 Third Avenue, New York, NY 10158

*Routledge is an imprint of the Taylor & Francis Group, an informa business*

*British Library Cataloguing-in-Publication Data*
A catalogue record for this book is available from the British Library

*Library of Congress Cataloging-in-Publication Data*
Names: Elliott, Alison (Senior lecturer in mental health), editor. |
Wright, Karen M., editor.
Title: Patient safety and serious incident responses : the essentials/ edited by Alison Elliott and Karen Wright.
Description: Abingdon, Oxon ; New York, NY : Routledge, 2025. |
Includes bibliographical references and index.
Identifiers: LCCN 2024026634 (print) | LCCN 2024026635 (ebook) |
ISBN 9781032260440 (hardback) | ISBN 9781032260426 (paperback) |
ISBN 9781003286240 (ebook)
Subjects: MESH: Patient Safety | Medical Errors | Safety Management
Classification: LCC R859.7.S43 (print) | LCC R859.7.S43 (ebook) |
NLM WX 185 | DDC 610.28/9—dc23/eng/20240618
LC record available at https://lccn.loc.gov/2024026634
LC ebook record available at https://lccn.loc.gov/2024026635

ISBN: 978-1-032-26044-0 (hbk)
ISBN: 978-1-032-26042-6 (pbk)
ISBN: 978-1-003-28624-0 (ebk)

DOI: 10.4324/9781003286240

Typeset in Times New Roman
by codeMantra

# Contents

# Figures

# Tables

# About the editors

**Alison Elliott**

Alison is a registered mental health nurse with over 40 years of experience in clinical practice and academia. Alison's clinical experience includes senior roles in acute mental health and older adult settings, but most of her experience has been in secure mental health and learning disability settings, managing and developing services. In her role at the University of Central Lancashire, she has been course leader for the BSc (Hons) Psychosocial Mental Health Care, MSc Personality Disorder, and PG Cert Investigating Serious Incidents, and programme lead for the Offender Personality Disorder Programme.

**Professor Karen M. Wright**

Karen Wright has a diverse range of clinical experience spanning more than 40 years. She has led and developed services, as well as nursing and psychotherapy curricula. She is a qualified nurse (Adult and Mental Health registrations), academic, and practicing psychotherapist and accredited member of the British Association of Cognitive Behavioural Psychotherapists. Karen is also chair of an NHS local research ethics committee. She recently retired from the University of Central Lancashire where she was Professor of Nursing, retaining an active Emeritus role.

# Contributors

**Kim Bennett** is a registered nurse with over 30 years' experience, the last ten of which have been within the field of patient safety and governance. Kim worked with Mersey Care on the implementation of the new Patient Safety Incident Response Framework.

**James Clapson** is a former British paratrooper and terrorism specialist, with 24 years of frontline operational experience in hostile environments across the Middle East, Europe, and Africa.

**David Durrant** has spent over 25 years working as a probation officer and, more recently, an operational manager within prisons. He currently commissions Offender Personality Disorder Services on behalf of His Majesty's Prison and Probation Service, in the South of England and Wales.

**Sue Ellis** is a retired training consultant, researcher, academic, and clinician.

**Louise Hamer** is Deputy Designated Nurse for Safeguarding Children and Children in Care at Lancashire and South Cumbria ICB. She is a children's nurse and health visitor.

**Julian Hendy** is an award-winning documentary filmmaker and investigative journalist. He is the founder of the Hundred Families charity, supporting families bereaved by homicides by people with severe mental illness. Hundred Families works across the UK with the NHS, Ministry of Justice, and others to prevent further tragedies and to promote lasting improvements in services. www.hundred-families.org

**Joanne Keeling** is the Associate Head of Postgraduate Taught Programmes in the School of Health Sciences at the University of Liverpool. Joanne is a registered mental health nurse.

**Teresa Lean** is a consultant nurse working for Lancashire and South Cumbria NHS Trust.

**Tim McDougall** is Executive Director of Quality, Nursing, and Healthcare Professionals at Pennine Care NHS Foundation Trust. Tim spent 15 years as a CAMHS nurse consultant and several as a clinical director in CAMHS and children's services.

**Dr Peggy Mulongo** is a cross-cultural mental health practitioner, lecturer, and researcher, with a focus on heath inequalities, race, and ethnicity. She has many years' experience of working with victims of female genital mutilation (FGM), gender-based violence, and domestic servitude in the North-West of England.

**Dr Jo Ramsden** is an NHS consultant clinical psychologist who works with people who have received or who could potentially attract the diagnosis of 'personality disorder'. Jo is particularly interested in the organisational conditions needed to support complex relational work.

**Dr Jenny Shaw** is a senior manager who has worked in the NHS, the independent sector, and higher education. She currently works with national and local incident investigation teams.

**Tiffany (Tiff) Sinclair** is a senior lecturer at the University of Central Lancashire.

**Louise Swarbrick** has a breadth of experience in a variety of settings, predominantly in the NHS. Louise has worked in a number of roles, including clinical nurse specialist in a specialist rehabilitation service, CMHT team manager and, more recently, clinical lead of an offender personality disorder service. With this varied experience, Louise has a nuanced understanding at leadership level of how change happens in complex systems.

**Dr John Wainwright** is the Director of the Global Race Centre for Equality (GRACE) at the University of Central Lancashire and has experience working with children, young people, and their families in the care and youth justice system.

**DCI Frankie Westoby** is a detective superintendent in the police service with nearly 30 years' operational policing experience within several forces and national units including the National Mental Health and Policing portfolio.

**Kevin Wright** is a senior lecturer at the University of Central Lancashire.

**Dr Panchu Xavier** is a consultant forensic psychiatrist with a high-security hospital. He is Deputy Chief Medical Officer for Quality and Patient Safety and Director of Patient Safety at a mental health and community trust in the North-West of England.

Valuable contributions were also made by following:

**Natalie Hammond** is Director of Nursing and Quality and an honorary professor who is passionate that improvements in healthcare are made through learning and prevention from safety incident analysis.

**Georgia Warne** is Associate Director of the Inquiry Project Team within Essex Partnership University NHS Foundation Trust (EPUT).

# Foreword

*Professor Mike Thomas*

A text which explores issues related to healthcare investigations, with a particular focus on safety incident response, has been needed, and wanted, for some time. This is because the primary function of all healthcare providers is to ensure the safety of users and carers whilst delivering the highest quality of care. And this care is relational, it is personal and human. Contemporary healthcare users have an expectation that they will be supported by health providers to be as independent as possible, to be provided with choices regarding their own care, and to have appropriate responses when their wellbeing is compromised.

Care remains a predominantly human interaction, even acknowledging the importance of technology in modern care, and behaviours, emotions, and communications interact simultaneously within individuals and groups. Inevitably, therefore, due to the interplay of human interactions, scrutiny is applied to the areas of healthcare safety, quality, and resources in attempts to gain assurance that predetermined standards of care are effective and caring, and carried out in a safe environment. Relevant regulatory frameworks are put in place, expected to be implemented, then externally tested regarding compliance and continuous improvement. (For example, the Care Quality Commission (CQC) carry out regular scrutiny of healthcare providers and publish their findings with the aim of creating a continuous learning environment within organisations.)

Healthcare providers and practitioners are required to have their own internal organisational processes and procedures to manage issues of safety, compliance and assurance, and carry out a root cause analysis (RCA) investigation where serious incidents occur. The investigation examines how and why an incident occurred, what lessons are learned to minimise reoccurrence, and what steps need to be implemented to provide improved safety. One can imagine the complexity involved. Will an investigation focus on human error, or relational and communications issues, behavioural or procedural issues, or the interplay between all of them? How does the investigation involve the end user, families, and carers? Should regulatory agencies be alerted, and when? What about afterwards – how are checks carried out to ensure learning has taken place? How is blame and retribution avoided so learning can be undertaken? How are the feelings of patients, users, families, and carers taken into account after an investigation? And where do kindness, compassion, and civility play a part? What are the issues that impact on the RCA investigation itself?

To have a text that examines safety incident response and investigations *beyond root cause analysis* is therefore welcome as it provides both exploration and guidance for such questions.

The text takes four sequential approaches. Part 1 examines the principles of investigations and, alongside procedural guidance, has an important contribution from Julian Hendy regarding family engagement. Part 2 explores issues when conducting the investigation, and in recognition of relational factors, Sue Ellis brings out the absolute importance of managing interpersonal dynamics. Part 3 brings various perspectives from different environments, such as custody settings and the military, when investigating cases involving children and families, and approaches needing cultural sensitivity. Part 4 delves into the issues that arise post-investigation and how to approach areas such as report presentations, executive summaries, and coroner's reports.

All the authors have personal experience of safety incidents investigations, sometimes not always positive, and bring a genuine sense of their lived experiences when addressing issues. Collectively, under the guidance of the editors, Alison and Karen, the chapter contributors provide a systematic, inclusive, consistent, and robust approach to safety incident responses and investigations. Crucially, the contributors stress the importance for healthcare providers and staff to *really* learn from safety incident responses and root cause analysis, and to do so within a culture that respects and embraces the values of compassion and kindness.

I hope you enjoy reading this important text and can apply the contents to your own environment.

# Acknowledgements

There are always too many people to mention when we reflect upon not only those who have contributed to the text but those who have influenced us in our journey to producing this text. We have both been influenced by people, organisations, and situations for many decades of practice and learning.

First, we would like to acknowledge those people who will be nameless but have been affected by events that we too have experienced in a multitude of roles. Maybe we were clinicians, observers, investigators, managers, family members or, indeed, victims. Maybe we did the right thing, maybe we stumbled through it, and maybe we still carry the scars ourselves?

The overwhelming factor that brought us to this point was a sense of responsibility to help others to 'get this right' – to enable them to approach their unique situation with the tools they need, with professionalism and with robust adherence to guidelines and protocols, and to be able to hold on to compassion and empathy for those affected. The people who enabled us to recognise this responsibility were our students on our academic programme (PGCert) at the University of Central Lancashire: *Dear Students, you have been our inspiration.*

To the chapter authors: thank you so much for sacrificing time and sleep to share your knowledge, insight, and wisdom.

To our families: our laptops are not really extensions of our arms… Thank you for bearing with us.

Alison and Karen

# Introduction

*Karen M. Wright and Alison Elliott*

In any environment providing care or a service to people, there is the possibility of adverse events (Kirkup, 2019), as can be seen by the plethora of investigations and inquiries going back decades, such as the Victoria Climbié Inquiry (Laming, 2003), the David 'Rocky' Bennett Inquiry (Blofeld et al., 2003), the Francis Report into the failures in Mid Staffordshire (2013), the inquiries undertaken into failures in maternity care in Morecambe Bay (Kirkup, 2015) and East Kent (Kirkup, 2019); not to mention the independent public inquiry led by Lady Justice Thirlwell to investigate the repeated failures that allowed neonatal nurse Lucy Letby to murder vulnerable infants in her care (Kirkup & Titcombe, 2023).

Practitioners, service users, and academics will appreciate the value of a robust and comprehensive inquiry, which seeks to elicit a deep understanding of events, without 'blame' (Radhakrishna, 2015). Although it has been stated that inquiries in relation to adverse events have become a standard response in the UK (Goodwin, 2018), it is also suggested that nurturing a 'culture of inquiry and learning' is important in relation to enhancing organisational performance and innovation (Alerasoul et al., 2022).

This book is as aimed at practitioners working in a variety of settings and promotes that sense of learning that should occur within, and because of, inquiry. In this text, we consider inquiry that seeks to investigate events and actions that have resulted in error, harm, malpractice, or neglect. To do this well, it is vital that we adopt an unbiased and enquiring approach and are led by robust protocols and guidance such as are described within this text, which also brings together a range of perspectives and professional disciplines.

We do not claim to have covered every possible aspect or issue that may arise within the context of the investigation of events or people, but we aim to provide transferable theories and models to guide the investigative process and, more importantly, to create learning which can transform practice as a result. For this, we suggest that a *culture of inquiry* is needed:

> A culture of inquiry is a safe, supportive space wherein practitioner-researchers are enabled to share their vulnerabilities, to make explicit their values, and to hold themselves accountable for living according to those values.
>
> (Vaughan & Delong, 2019: 65)

DOI: 10.4324/9781003286240-1

This is no mean feat when something has gone badly wrong and requires investigation and a determination to do things differently in the future; blame, accusations, and fear may abound. Such inquiries are often pivotal turning points in terms of health policy and practice. For example, following the inquiry into the high mortality rate in children who had undergone cardiac surgery in Bristol in the 1990s (Kennedy, 2002), the Commission for Health Improvement was established, with the aim of developing clinical governance and supporting healthcare organisations to improve their quality of service to patients (Benson et al., 2006). The inquiries into the crimes of Beverley Allitt (Clothier, 1994) and Harold Shipman (Smith, 2002) both had significant impacts in terms of healthcare professionals' regulation (Quick, 2014).

Sadly, it often takes things to go wrong to bring us to a point of realisation that we need to change. How we need to change may be revealed through an investigation, although many of us will have experienced that overwhelming sense of *what* needs to change long before an investigation/inquiry has been conducted or its findings published, and will have experienced a multitude of emotions and thoughts that may interrupt our daily existence in the meantime. Historical cases such as those mentioned above led to changes to professional regulation and have been turning points. Indeed, clinical governance in the NHS was developed in response to an apparent need and is defined as:

> a system through which NHS organisations are accountable for continuously improving the quality of their services and safeguarding high standards of care by creating an environment in which excellence in clinical care will flourish.
>
> (NHS England, 2021: 12)

Ultimately, the systems and processes underpinned by clinical governance are intended to underpin mechanisms for ensuring patient safety and quality. Other organisations will have their own, all aligning to such principles. However, despite the tidal changes that stemmed from historical cases, and the focus on patient safety from 2000 onwards, and despite senior practitioners being to be trained in the use of root cause analysis (RCA) in an attempt to instigate a standardised approach to investigation of adverse events, it is clear that the continued system failures mean we still have much to learn. Martin-Delgado and colleagues explain that:

> RCA is a useful tool for the identification of the remote and immediate causes of safety incidents, but not for implementing effective measures to prevent their recurrence.
>
> (Martin-Delgado et al., 2020: 254)

Hence, merely discovering *why* things have happened results in the same old recommendations being rolled out, simply to be ignored, as is demonstrated by reports detailing similar recommendations and accompanied by a strong sense of déjà vu. Lists of advice to provide supervision, training, and so on create box-ticking exercises, effectively blaming those responsible and implicitly saying that they need greater overseeing and informing. Indeed, Kellogg et al. (2016) wondered if RCA had actually contributed to failures to improve patient safety. This text does not focus on RCA, as there are plenty of others that do; rather, it focuses on more contemporary approaches that seek to make a difference and include those affected in the process.

Many inquiries evoke a gamut of emotions, reinforced by media coverage, but when the BBC *Panorama* documentary exposed not only neglectful and cruel practice but also the toxic culture within Edenfield hospital, it was clear that we had learned little from the Francis Inquiry (2013). It will be interesting to see the outcomes of the inquiry into the case of Lucy Letby, the neonatal nurse at the Countess of Chester Hospital who was found guilty of killing seven babies and attempting to kill a further six between June 2015 and June 2016.

The introduction of the Patient Safety Incident Response Framework (NHS England, 2022) provided a much-needed, more sophisticated understanding and alternative approaches to investigation, with an acknowledgement that the complexity of healthcare environments required practitioners to be able to access a 'toolbox' of approaches to investigation, such as the consideration of 'human factors' (Brennan et al., 2022) and 'systems theory' (Lounsbury & Sujan, 2023). We argue that these approaches are transferable to other complex environments and situations and that they need to maintain a 'culture of inquiry' rather than an 'inquiry culture', so that a 'just' and learning culture can be maintained and those affected can be treated fairly and compassionately.

This text is organised somewhat chronologically in terms of the process of inquiry, but also brings together a range of perspectives and professional disciplines to discusses the process of investigation in a variety of settings, with evidence-based techniques/approaches that we hope will be useful to practitioners – especially those undertaking investigations in addition to their 'day job'.

The use of evidence-based, tried-and-tested approaches means that ethical principles and justice can be served, and that the victims (and second victims) of serious incidents are treated with respect and have their rights addressed in the search for truth, and, we hope, that such investigations produce meaningful, achievable, proportionate, and – most importantly – effective outcomes.

## References

Alerasoul, S. A., Afeltra, G., Hakala, H., Minelli, E., & Strozzi, F. (2022). Organisational learning, learning organisation, and learning orientation: An integrative review and framework. *Human Resource Management Review*, 32(3), 100854–100860.

Benson, L. A., Boyd, A., & Walshe, K. (2006). Learning from regulatory interventions in healthcare: The Commission for Health Improvement and its clinical governance review process. *Clinical Governance*, 11(3), 213–224.

Blofeld, J., Sallah, D., Sashidharan, S., Stone, R., & Struthers, J. (2003). *Independent inquiry into the death of David Bennett*. Norfolk, Suffolk and Cambridgeshire Strategic Health Authority.

Brennan, P. A., Jarvis, S., & Oeppen, R. S. (2022). European Association of Oral Medicine 2021 Conference – Crispian Scully Lecture: Applying Human Factors to Improve Patient Safety and Performance. *Journal of Oral Pathology & Medicine*, 51(1), 13–17.

Clothier, C. (1994). *The Allitt inquiry: Independent inquiry relating to deaths and injuries on the children's ward at Grantham and Kesteven General Hospital during the period February to April 1991.* London: HMSO.

Francis, R. (2013). *Report of the Mid Staffordshire NHS Trust Public Inquiry – Executive Summary.* London: The Stationery Office.

Goodwin, D. (2018). Cultures of caring: Healthcare 'scandals', inquiries, and the remaking of accountabilities. *Social Studies of Science*, 48(1), 101–124.

Kellogg, K. M., Hettinger, Z., Shah, M., Wears, R. L., Sellers, C. R., Squires, M., & Fairbanks, R. J. (2016). Our current approach to root cause analysis: Is it contributing to our failure to improve patient safety? *BMJ Quality & Safety*, 26(5), 381–387.

Kennedy, I. (Chair) (2002). *The Report of the Public Inquiry into Children's Heart Surgery at the Bristol Royal Infirmary 1984–1995.* London: The Stationery Office.

Kirkup, B. (2015). The impact of the Kirkup report. *Midwives*, 18(2), 51.

Kirkup, B. (2019). NHS Improvement's Just Culture Guide: Good intentions failed by flawed design. *Journal of the Royal Society of Medicine*, 112(12), 495–497.

Kirkup, B., & Titcombe, J. (2023). Patient safety: Listen to whistleblowers. *BMJ: British Medical Journal (Online)*, 382, 1972. Available from: www.proquest.com/scholarly-journals/patient-safety-listen-whistleblowers/docview/2859292617/se-2.

Laming, W. H. (2003). *The Victoria Climbié inquiry: Report of an inquiry by Lord Laming* (Cm. 5730). London: The Stationery Office.

Lounsbury, O., & Sujan, M. (2023). Achieving a restorative Just Culture through the patient safety incident response framework. *Journal of Patient Safety and Risk Management*, 28(4), 153–155.

Martin-Delgado, J., Martínez-García, A., Aranaz, J. M., Valencia-Martín, J. L., & Mira, J. J. (2020). How much of root cause analysis translates into improved patient safety: A systematic review. *Medical Principles and Practice*, 29(6), 524–531.

NHS England. (2021). *The matron's handbook.* Available from: www.england.nhs.uk/wp-content/uploads/2021/07/Matrons-Handbook-July-2021.pdf

NHS England. (2022). *Patient Safety Incident Response Framework (PSIRF) and supporting guidance.* London: NHS England.

Quick, O. (2014). Regulating and legislating safety: The case for candour. *BMJ Quality & Safety*, 23(8), 614–618.

Radhakrishna, S. (2015). Culture of blame in the National Health Service: Consequences and solutions. *BJA: British Journal of Anaesthesia*, 115(5), 653–655.

Smith, J. (2002). *The Shipman Inquiry first report.* Available from: https://webarchive.nationalarchives.gov.uk/ukgwa/20090808160147/http://www.the-shipman-inquiry.org.uk/firstreport.asp

Vaughan, M., & Delong, J. (2019). Cultures of inquiry: A transformative method of creating living-theories. *Educational Journal of Living Theories*, 12(2), 65.

# PART 1
# Principles of investigation

# 1 Understanding and avoiding unconscious bias

*Alison Elliott*

Investigations in health and social care settings are important and complex processes, and are essential for organisational learning, however the quality of an investigation is largely dependent on the interpersonal effectiveness, self-awareness, knowledge, and skills of the investigator (Binns & Sachman, 2020). This chapter will discuss the pivotal role that the investigator plays in any investigation, and the need for them to be aware of their own unconscious/implicit and explicit biases, so that those involved in the investigation are treated fairly and equitably.

The 2023 case of Lucy Letby, the neonatal nurse convicted of murdering seven babies and attempting to kill at least six others at the Countess of Chester Hospital, is a devastating example of a failure to investigate the concerns raised by whistle-blowers, who were not only accused of bullying her (and required to apologise), but were also threatened with being reported to the General Medical Council. Such a failure to act by those responsible will be explored by the statutory inquiry; however, as with other cases of medical professionals causing harm, there were missed opportunities to stop Letby.

It has been suggested that the 'top-down' culture in the NHS means that senior managers are preoccupied by reputation, and that more junior managers feel obliged to maintain an impression that *all is well*, even if the opposite is true (Mathew, 2023). Whilst this may have been the case with Letby, rare but repeated cases of medical/nursing professionals causing harm suggests that stereotypes of doctors/nurses (Rudland & Mires, 2005) and assumptions about behaviour and conduct may have been a factor in the failure to investigate in the Letby case.

Serious incident investigations are therefore essential if organisations are to learn from adverse events, and eliciting and understanding the perspectives of those involved is a vital but challenging part of the process (Kok et al., 2022). At the beginning of this process, the key informants must be identified (see Chapter 5) and should include those practitioners directly involved in any incident itself, as well as patients, families, and carers affected, as they are likely to have different knowledge and information from that of professionals (Birkeland, 2019). According to Van Dael et al. (2022), who analysed five years' worth of patient complaints and staff incident reports at a large hospital in London, in areas where there was an overlap between complaints and incidents, there were significantly higher rates of incidents and potential for serious harm. This supports the notion that the

DOI: 10.4324/9781003286240-3

involvement of family and carers (see Chapter 4) in investigations is essential due to their insights in relation to service delivery, as is the need for their contribution to be valued and used to inform organisational learning and improvement, and to avoid 'epistemic injustice', described by Fricker (2009) as the devaluing of another's knowledge due to the prejudice of the hearer.

Most trained investigators are senior practitioners, therefore enabling a possible power imbalance in investigatory processes, and reinforcing the need for an open, non-judgemental and transparent approach (Kok et al., 2022) to support a rigorous and comprehensive investigation. This is especially true when an incident has occurred due to the human error of a colleague:

> Thinking through error trajectories, devising questions with which to approach colleagues involved in the error, speculating about causes and deciding on and formulating recommendations are all very loaded processes, particularly if people from 'the department in question' are on the RCA team.
>
> (Iedema et al., 2006: 1607)

The need to be inclusive (see Chapter 9) and to value the experiences and perspectives of a variety of informants during the investigatory process illustrates the need for the investigator to take an informed facilitative approach to the investigation.

**Self-awareness** and the ability to establish a rapport with a diverse range of people, using an appropriate investigation methodology or approach is vital (Astill, 2008; Bhandari et al., 2022) to establish a helpful relationship with informants in which they feel able to share their experiences and perspectives, and to enable an inclusive and equitable approach. Hence, investigators need to maintain an awareness of their own unconscious/implicit and explicit biases.

**Implicit bias**, also referred to as 'unconscious bias', is described by Kruse (2015) as the positive or negative preferences for individuals, groups, or things that have been shaped by our individual life experiences, family, and peers. Explicit biases are our preferences for people, things, and groups that we are consciously aware of (but may not share if we are aware reactions to them may be negative), also shaped by our family and peer influences, and life experiences. It has been suggested that our capacity to categorise everyone and everything we encounter is an evolutionary development that ensured our survival as it enabled judgements to be made in relation to danger (Banaji & Greenwald, 2013). Both implicit and explicit biases are important as humans are prone to make judgements or assumptions about others based on scant information, such as brief descriptions of single characteristics or behaviours (Torodov & Uleman, 2002), or facial characteristics (Rule et al., 2010), which is important as once these initial inferences have been activated, they tend to persist (Shoda et al., 2014). Implicit bias can also have a significant impact on non-verbal communication such as posture and levels of eye contact, and therefore adversely impact on interpersonal relationships and communication (De Paulo & Friedman, 1998; Hamilton & Stroessner, 2021), which has the potential to adversely impact the quality and depth of an investigation.

Implicit bias is also inextricably linked to stereotypes and stigma – the social consequences of negative attributions (Pilgrim, 2017) – which influence the quality of an investigation and play a key role in how clinicians care for and treat service users and their fellow professionals, highlighting both the complexity of the dynamics of interpersonal relationships and investigations (Fitzgerald & Hurst, 2017).

**Stereotypes**, or 'automatic associations' (Hamilton & Stroessner, 2021), are the beliefs held in relation to the generally negative qualities and characteristics of specific groups or individuals. These negative stereotypes then evoke emotions such as contempt, disgust, and fear, although occasionally other emotions such as pity can be elicited (Pilgrim, 2017). Such stereotypes can be linked to stigma and discrimination, and if held by an investigator who is unaware of them, will adversely impact on their capacity to take an inclusive and fair approach. They may also stigmatise and therefore discount the importance of some of those with pertinent information in relation to the investigation. Stigma and stereotypes can have a powerful impact on how we treat others – for example, at the start of the human immunodeficiency virus (HIV) pandemic, many clinicians assumed that the virus was confined to the gay community, which provoked further stigma and discrimination and meant that recognition of wider transmission to other communities was delayed (Marcelin et al., 2019).

In an investigation, bias, stereotyping, and stigma can be mitigated by the investigator being self-aware and reflective, and by ensuring that they take a fair and equitable approach to all relevant persons involved. Marcelin et al. (2019) would suggest that this awareness of one's own biases, being transparent in decision making and following relevant guidelines, as well as being open to learning about others and new experiences means that they can be addressed before they impact on others, ensuring that a consistently fair, respectful, and equitable approach can be maintained. They also suggest that if bias does occur, its effects can be mitigated if practitioners (and investigators) own their actions, consider the experience of others, ensure that they actively seek to rebuild trust and self-reinforce behaviours that will prevent recurrence.

In addition to self-awareness and awareness of stereotypes, stigma, and their impact, investigators must ensure that they recognise the importance of a 'just and learning culture' (NHS England & NHS Improvement, 2019), first suggested in the seminal *An Organisation with a Memory* (Department of Health, 2000), and described as:

> A just culture: not a total absence of blame, but an atmosphere of trust in which people are encouraged to provide safety related information, at the same time being clear about where the line is drawn between acceptable and unacceptable behaviours.
>
> (Department of Health, 2000: 35)

This therefore presents investigators (and leaders) with a challenge as this 'just culture' focuses on the development of a blame-free culture as recommended by the Being Open Framework (National Patient Safety Agency (NPSA), 2009) in relation to adverse events, and understanding how systems and human factors may have influenced events; however, this has been the opposite of the experiences of many practitioners who have been involved in such investigations (Tingle, 2021) (see Chapter 17).

It is essential, therefore, that investigators can use effective communication and a compassionate and inclusive approach, as a serious incident is traumatic for all affected (MacDonald et al., 2014), and compassionate approaches have been shown to enhance wellbeing (de Zulueta, 2021). Communication models such as SOLER (Egan, 1975) could support this ('**S**it squarely'; '**O**pen posture'; '**L**ean towards the other'; '**E**ye contact'; '**R**elax'); however, other issues such as consideration of where interviews take place, whether to use group or individual interviews, whether the support of translators or administrative staff is needed, how much time is required and whether the interviewee would need additional support (from a colleague or their union representative) are all also important and are discussed in subsequent chapters.

Given the significant impact of serious incidents, a compassionate leadership approach is important for investigators in accordance with the principles of Being Open (NPSA, 2009), as the stress experienced can be far-reaching and long-lasting, and, for practitioners, have a significant impact on their practice (MacDonald et al., 2014). This compassionate and collaborative approach to undertaking investigations is reinforced by the recently published *Patient Safety Investigation Standards* (NHS England, 2022) in which a strategic, preventative (investigations are conducted to support learning and prevent recurrence), collaborative, fair and just, people-focused, credible, trustworthy, and adept (conducted by teams with requisite expertise) approach is required, with staff being active and supported participants.

This shift links to the current paradigm in relation to patient safety and the investigation of incidents, in that rather than focusing on what went wrong (a Safety-I approach), there is a focus on a Safety-II approach (Mannion & Braithwaite, 2017), in which there is an emphasis on what has been done well, as this also enables consideration and understanding as to what may have gone wrong. Given that the Safety-I approach does not seem to have yielded change, as many investigations repeatedly have the same findings and make similar recommendations, the appreciative approach of Safety-II would seem to offer possibilities, provided the issues in relation to Safety-I are also addressed. Worldwide, there are issues in relation to patient safety (World Health Organization, 2017); however, despite this, and the fact that organisations are required to have incident-reporting systems in place, such incidents are often underreported (Sari et al., 2007), rarely acted upon (Jha & Pronovost, 2016) and poorly investigated (Smith & Valenta, 2018), as practitioners are not routinely trained in a variety of approaches, and therefore meaningful change in relation to compensatory action rarely takes place (Carson-Stevens et al., 2018). In the UK, the Patient Safety Incident Response Framework (NHS England, 2022) represents an opportunity to address these issues, if implemented consistently, and taking an appreciative approach that focuses on what has been done well should create an environment where practitioners feel more able to share their perspectives and experiences. It has also been suggested that this may be more compatible with the complexities of healthcare environments as it does not use the 'cause equals effect' approach of Safety-I (Braithwaite et al., 2015).

However, there may well be occasions where a Safety-I approach is required – for example, failures/faulty equipment or sustained deviation from policies and procedures – as it has been estimated that in 2012 around 40 per cent of care was not delivered in accordance with recommended or evidence-based practice (Runciman et al, 2012), and given the demands of the current healthcare landscape, it would appear that this has not improved (Smaggus, 2019). In this case, a self-aware investigator with a compassionate approach and sound interpersonal skills using an evidence-based approach to investigation will be more likely to be able to elicit information from those directly involved. Additionally, beyond the investigation, sound interpersonal skills are imperative to enable them to gain acceptance by their colleagues during the aftermath of the investigation to enable learning and change (Iedema et al., 2006).

To conclude, the quality of an investigation, whether using a Safety-I or a Safety-II approach is fundamentally influenced by the attitudes, biases, and values of the investigator, as well as their level of training and seniority. However, an awareness of such attitudes, biases, and values can be developed via training in unconscious bias, by reflection, by testing (Implicit Attitude Test; Greenwald et al., 1998) and by ongoing supervision. This awareness is related to the need for 'critical consciousness', described by Freire (1993) as an appreciation that we do not exist in isolation, and that knowledge and culture are ever changing. This illustrates the need for investigators to be critical thinkers and to engage in critical self-reflection, described as:

> not a singular focus on the self, but a stepping back to understand one's own assumptions, biases and values and a shifting of one's gaze from oneself to others.
>
> (Kumagai and Lypson, 2009: 783)

## References

Astill, D. (2008). Ensuring optimal learning from adverse incidents: the importance of a robust serious untoward incident investigation. *Clinical Risk*, 14(1): 18–20.

Banaji, M. R., & Greenwald, A. G. (2013). *Blindspot: Hidden Biases of Good People* (1st ed.). New York, NY: Delacorte Press.

Bhandari, S., Thomassen, O., & Nathan, R. (2022). Causation, historiographic approaches and the investigation of serious adverse incidents in mental health settings. *Health*, 27(6), 1019–1032.

Binns, C., & Sachman, B. (eds). (2020). *The Art of Investigation*. Boco Raton, FL: CRC Press.

Birkeland, S. (2019). Healthcare complaints and adverse events as a means of user involvement for quality and safety improvement. *The Millbank Quarterly*, 97(1), 346–349.

Braithwaite, J., Wears, R.L., & Hollnagel, E. (2015). Resilient health care: Turning patient safety on its head. *International Journal for Quality in Health Care*, 27(5), 418–420.

Carson-Stevens, A., Donaldson, L., & Sheikh, A. (2018). The rise of Patient Safety-II: Should we give up hope on Safety-I and extracting value from patient safety incidents? *International Journal of Health Policy and Management*, 7(7), 667–670.

Department of Health. (2000). *An Organisation with a Memory: Report of an Expert Group on Learning from Adverse Events in the NHS Chaired by the Chief Medical Officer*. London: The Stationery Office.

De Paulo, B. M., & Friedman, H. S. (1998). Nonverbal communication. In: Gilbert D.T., Fiske, & S.T., Lindzey, G (eds). *The Handbook of Social Psychology*, Vol. 2 (4th ed.) New York; McGraw-Hill, 3–40.

de Zulueta, P. (2021). How do we sustain compassionate healthcare? Compassionate leadership in the time of the COVID-19 pandemic. *Clinics in Integrated Care*, 8, 100071.

Egan, G. (1975). *The Skilled Helper: A Systematic Approach to Effective Helping*. Pacific Grove, CA: Brooks/Cole.

Fitzgerald, C., & Hurst, S. (2017). Implicit bias in healthcare professionals: A systematic review. *BMC Medical Ethics*, 18(19), 1–18.

Freire, P. (1993). *Pedagogy of the Oppressed* (20th anniversary ed.). New York, NY: Continuum.

Fricker, M. (2009). *Epistemic Injustice. Power and the Ethics of Knowing.* Oxford University Press.

Greenwald, A. G., McGhee, D. E., & Schwartz, J. L. (1998). Measuring individual differences in implicit cognition: the implicit association test. *Journal of Personal and Social Psychology*, 74, 1464–1480.

Hamilton, D. L., & Stroessner, S. J. (2021). *Social Cognition; Understanding People and Events*. Sage Publications.

Iedema, R. A. M., Jorm, C., Long, D., Braithwaite, J., Travaglia, J., & Westbrook, M. (2006). Turning the medical gaze in upon itself: Root cause analysis and the investigation of clinical error. *Social Science & Medicine*, 62(7), 1605–1615.

Jha, A., & Pronovost, P. (2016). Toward a safer health care system: The critical need to improve measurement. *JAMA*, 315(17), 1831–1832.

Kok, J., de Kam, D., Leistikow, I., Grit, K., & Bal, R. (2022). Epistemic justice in incident investigations: A qualitative study. *Health Care Analysis*, 30, 254–274. https://doi.org/10.1007/s10728-022-00447-3

Kruse, C. (2015). Unconscious bias: 3 key steps to help organisations successfully address the issue. *Personal Excellence Essentials*, 20(1), 20–26.

Kumagai, A. K., & Lypson, M. L. (2009). Beyond cultural competence: Critical consciousness, social justice, and multicultural education. *Academic Medicine*, 84(6), 782–787.

MacDonald, M., Gosakan, R., Cooper, A. E., & Fothergill, D. J. (2014). Dealing with a serious incident requiring investigation in obstetrics and gynaecology: A training perspective. *The Obstetrician & Gynaecologist*, 16, 109–114.

Mannion, R., & Braithwaite, J. (2017). False dawns and new horizons in patient safety research and practice. *International Journal of Health Policy Management*, 6(12), 685–689.

Marcelin, J. R., Siraj, D. S., Victor, R., Kotadia, S., & Maldonado, Y. A. (2019). The impact of unconscious bias in healthcare: How to recognise it and mitigate it. *The Journal of Infectious Diseases*, 220(Suppl. 2), 62–73.

Mathew, R. (2023). Taking stock: Lucy Letby and the limits of a no blame culture. *BMJ*, 382, 1966.

National Patient Safety Agency (2009). *Being Open: Saying Sorry When Things Go Wrong.* London: NPSA.

NHS England/NHS Improvement. (2019). *The NHS Patient Safety Strategy: Safer culture, safer systems, safer patients.* London: NHS England/NHS Improvement.

NHS England. (2022). *Patient Safety Incident Response Framework (PSIRF) and supporting guidance.* London: NHS England.

Pilgrim, D. (2017). *Key Concepts in Mental Health* (4th ed.). Sage Publications.

Rudland, J. R., & Mires, G. J. (2005). Characteristics of doctors and nurses as perceived by students entering medical school: Implications for shared teaching. *Medical Education,* 39(5), 448–455.

Rule, N., Ambady, N., Adams, R., Ozono, H., Nakashima, S., Yoshikawa, S., & Watabe, M. (2010). Polling the face: Prediction and consensus across cultures. *Journal of Personality and Social Psychology,* 98, 1–15.

Runciman, W. B., Hunt, T. D., Hannaford, N. A., Hibbert, P. D., Westbrook, J. I., Coiera, E. W., Day, R. O., Hindmarsh, D. M., McGlynn, E. A., & Braithwaite, J. (2012). CareTrack: assessing the appropriateness of health care delivery in Australia. *Medical Journal of Australia,* 197, 549.

Sari, A. B., Sheldon, T. A., Cracknell, A., & Turnbull, A. A. (2007). Sensitivity of routine system for reporting patient safety incidents in an NHS hospital: Retrospective patient case note review. *British Medical Journal,* 334(7584), 79.

Shoda, T. M., McConnell, A. R., & Rydell, R. J. (2014). Implicit consistency processes in social cognition: Explicit-implicit discrepancies across systems of evaluation. *Social and Personality Psychology Compass,* 8(3), 135–146.

Smaggus, A. (2019). Safety-I, Safety-II and burnout: How complexity science can help clinician wellness. *BMJ Quality & Safety,* 28(8), 667–671.

Smith, K. M., & Valenta, A. I. (2018). Safety I to Safety II: A paradigm shift or more work as imagined? *International Journal of Health Policy and Management,* 7(7), 671–673.

Tingle, J. (2021). Developing a just culture in the NHS. *British Journal of Nursing,* 3, 500–502.

Todorov, A., & Uleman, J. (2002). Spontaneous trait inferences are bound to actors' faces: Evidence from a false recognition paradigm. *Journal of Personality and Social Psychology,* 83(5), 105–1065.

Van Dael, J., Gillespie, A., Reader, T., Smalley, K., Papdimitriou, D., Glampson, B., Marshall, D., & Mayer, E. (2022). Getting the whole story: Integrating patient complaints and staff reports of unsafe care. *Journal of Health Services Research and Policy,* 27(1), 41–49.

World Health Organization. (2017). *Patient Safety: Making Health Care Safer.* Geneva: World Health Organization.

## Resources

Harvard Implicit Attitudes Test. Available from: https://implicit.harvard.edu/implicit/takeatest.html

NHS Employers Just and Learning Culture Information. Available from: www.nhsemployers.org/system/files/2021-07/Just%20and%20Learning%20Culture%20Information%20Jan2021.pdf

NHS England Just Culture Guide. Available from: www.england.nhs.uk/patient-safety/patient-safety-culture/a-just-culture-guide

# 2 To debrief or not to debrief

*Frankie Westoby*

Insanity is doing the same thing over and over and expecting different results.

Author unknown

## Introduction

The origins of debriefing are from the military, policing, and the aviation industry, although over the years the process of debriefing has been adopted more broadly across many other organisations (Hawker et al., 2011). Debriefing is a term that covers a variety of different functions and can vary within and between individuals and organisations. The move towards a learning culture both by individuals and organisations has seen the increased use of and development of several debriefing methods (Hebles et al., 2023). Most methods have links to the 'experiential learning cycle' framework developed by David Kolb, which focuses on the theory that learning through experience creates the knowledge (Kurt, 2022).

On a small scale, individuals may carry out personal reflection on a daily basis, considering how the day has gone or their individual response to an incident or event that has taken place. This kind of process enables self-learning and development, as suggested by Dewey (1916), more than a hundred years ago:

> The material of thinking is not thoughts, but actions, facts, events, and the relations of things. In other words, to think effectively one must have had, or now have experiences which will furnish … resources for coping with the difficulty at hand.

Dewey (2016: 156)

Following a significant incident or event for any organisation, there is the opportunity to debrief and learn from the incident. This chapter will focus on debriefing from the aspect of capturing organisational learning and the importance of taking the learning forward so that organisationally the same practice is not continually repeated and the outcome does change.

DOI: 10.4324/9781003286240-4

## The purpose of debriefing

Debriefing has several purposes. Fundamentally, its purpose is to identify good practice and areas for improvement in a psychologically safe and positive environment. Historically, debriefing grew from critical incidents that were thought to provoke stress in an individual. This has since developed and is now also used in simulation and education training (Edwards et al., 2021).

Psychological safety is very important if the true benefits of debriefing are to be realised, because if an individual partaking in a group debrief believes there is an element of blame, they may not engage, and the value of the debrief will be lost (Kolbe et al., 2020).

There are additional purposes of debriefing – for instance, debriefing emergency services, in some form of 'hot debrief', described by Sugerman et al. as 'a structured team-based discussion which may be initiated following a significant event' (2021: 579), usually immediately after (e.g. regarding the entry route into a scene, and activities that have taken place within) as this may have a consequential impact on an investigation and is important for investigative bodies to understand. Consideration is given to questions such as 'Has potential evidence been unavoidably disturbed or contaminated?' This sort of consideration has been relevant for several multi-agency major incidents in recent years, such as the 2017 Manchester Arena attack, the 2018 Novichok poisoning in Salisbury, and the 2019 London Bridge attack; this is a form of debrief but is not about organisational learning at the time, although it may become part of a more formal debrief process such as a structured debrief in the future.

Debriefing is regularly discussed as good practice but is not routinely completed (Gougoulis et al., 2020). There are many reasons for this, particularly in reference to blue light responders. The ability to debrief is often hampered due to the immediacy of the next incident and the inability to make time for debrief. In other areas, such as healthcare, the debrief itself may demand considerable skill and the lack of trained facilitators and guidelines becomes a barrier to widespread practice of debrief implementation (Healy & Tyrell, 2013). What is clear is that debriefing does not take place consistently across blue light services and health services (Omar et al., 2023). Furthermore, when it does happen, evidence shows it is often completed using untrained facilitators, which has the consequence of not ensuring that the best opportunities for learning are captured or that the learning is progressed (Cheng et al., 2021).

This inconsistent approach is at odds with best practice detailed by many organisations that suggests briefing, debriefing, and team preparation are advocated as best practice to optimise team and organisational performance (Edwards et al., 2018).

Debriefing is usually considered after a significant or major incident, but debriefing can be and should be used far more broadly, particularly if an organisation is focusing on creating a learning culture (Firing et al., 2020). Ensuring the use of debriefing validates the experience, helps clarify areas of misunderstanding or misconception and identifies areas for improvement. Debriefs can be utilised to capture the learning from adverse significant events and organisational change (Feuer, 2021), as well as environmental impacts, such as localised flooding, and simulated learning experiences, which in the author's experience are an important strategy in relation to multi-agency learning and service development.

## Types of debrief

Before a debrief is commenced, there is a need for clarity regarding the purpose of the debrief. There are many debrief models, and it is important to ensure that the appropriate model is used (Colleen et al., 2021). Questions should be asked such as whether the debrief is aimed at debriefing an incident or change, or whether it is a stress debrief which is focused more on debriefing emotions and on an individual's psychological welfare (Zigmont et al., 2011). It is important to make the distinction, so that participants understand the purpose of their involvement, and equally important to debrief good practice, to enhance organisational learning.

Incident debriefing processes should be incorporated into the daily business of blue light responders and other healthcare organisations (Neeley et al., 2023). The outcomes of creating such an environment enhance corporate knowledge and develop the expertise of staff involved. This is particularly relevant in emergencys or major incidents when several agencies could be involved (College of Policing, 2022b). This could be through a simple, short hot debrief taking a matter of minutes or a more structured approach taking several hours.

The fire service utilise the **hot debrief** method along with those working within emergency medicine. Developed in Edinburgh by Walker et al. (2020), the 'STOP5' framework aims to improve patient care following an incident in the emergency department. The first stage is to establish the wellbeing of everyone in the team, then to go on to the following points:

- **S**ummarise the case
- **T**hings that went well
- **O**pportunities to improve
- **P**oints to action and responsibilities.

This approach has been found to have overwhelmingly positive feedback, as staff reported that certain cases, particularly resuscitation cases, are emotionally challenging, and being able to stop and debrief enhanced wellbeing, together with the support the team were able to provide to each other (Scott et al., 2022).

Other organisations would benefit from taking the time to perform a hot debrief and the beneficial impact this process has on staff; however, time is often the disabling factor in that retaining staff after a shift to go through the process of a debrief can result in a lack of engagement. Timing is key to the success of any debrief process (Colleen et al, 2021).

Essex Police have recently developed a **rapid debrief process** for incidents of homicide and serious violence, which is a hybrid of the hot debrief and structured debrief process, and enables targeted preventative action to reduce the number of homicides (College of Policing, 2022a).

**Structured debriefing**, developed by the College of Policing, is a formal debrief process that can last several hours; it takes place some time after the incident and works to the terms of reference being requested by the senior leader for the incident. A questionnaire is circulated prior to the debrief, which assists the facilitator, scribe, and those attending the debrief as it enables the participants to reflect on the incident before attending the debrief. When the participants come together, consistent with other debrief processes, it aims to provide the psychologically safe and positive environment of other processes. Structured Debriefing works through a simple model of 'what went well', 'what didn't go so well', and 'considerations and learning going forward' in line with Kolb's experiential learning cycle (1984), and it encourages the participants to reflect on the concrete experience and modify and draw conclusions from the experience (College of Policing 2022a). Structured Debriefing is a well-tested process and has been used considerably to debrief multi-agency incidents across the UK in recent years (Grubb et al., 2021).

What has been disappointing is the lack of follow-up on the recommendations coming from such debriefs. Often the debrief is completed and that is seen as the final tick in the box, rather than acknowledging the learning, good practice, and areas for improvement being taken forward. There are small pockets of good practice where processes have been developed to track and take learning forward, Greater Manchester Police have a well-established process which was brought in after the Manchester Arena attack. From a multi-agency perspective, there has been the creation of the **Joint Organisational Learning (JOL)** hub on ResilienceDirect To ensure a learning culture going forward, all agencies across the country need to take responsibility for sharing learning and taking recommendations forward to encourage closer interoperability between blue light responders and other public services (Charman, 2014).

Like the structured debrief process, healthcare's debrief process for simulation-based medical training follows a similar model. It also includes a focus on the human factors. This process takes place immediately after an incident and therefore has a focus on emotions. It is a unique opportunity to come to an understanding about what happened and delve into the lessons learnt to influence and improve performance in the future (Gardner, 2013).

**Reflective debriefing** is used within healthcare settings and is a process that enables the participants to reflect on the incident and embrace critical thinking and learning for improving practice in the future (Hawkins, 2022). It is particularly useful for those who have less experience and incorporates mindfulness techniques to assist in building resilience whilst learning from the incident. This type of debrief is now being taken forward in the policing environment utilising Gibbs' Model of Reflection (Gibbs, 1988), recognising that the work force is currently very young and inexperienced and that working through the following areas can assist with learning:

- Description of the experience
- Thoughts and feelings about the experience
- Evaluating the experience (similar to structured debriefing)
- Analysis to enable some sense to be made of the incident

- Conclusions in relation to the areas learned, both positive and what would have been done differently
- A form of action plan or recommendations as to how to deal with similar incidents/events in the future.

Other forms of debrief include serious case reviews, multi-agency debrief, written debriefs and many more. The majority focus on what went well, areas for improvement, and the acknowledegment of good practice and recommendations going forward (Allen et al., 2018). There has been a move to terming recommendations as considerations, due to the nature of how the learning comes about within a debrief. It is for those present in the debrief, who were part of the event, to highlight the learning or consideration as they see it, and once the learning has been collated, for the recommendations to be developed and agreed by those reviewing.

There are some clear distinctions between debriefs in the healthcare setting and those of blue light responders. The health sector debrief processes tend to have a focus on emotions and human factors within the debrief process, whereas blue light debriefs tend to separate these processes (Allen et al., 2018). Blue light responders use bespoke debriefing models to support emotional wellbeing, and although these models are used in healthcare, there are some significant benefits to recognising emotions and human factors within the debrief, rather than separating them out. Trauma risk management (TRiM) (Greenberg at al., 2008) has been developed from clinical research, showing that most individuals who live through a traumatic incident adapt and adjust well with no long-term ill effects. The TRiM process enables those who are trained to deliver the debrief process to identify the difference between those individuals' displaying symptoms of acute stress that are normal and those who may need immediate referral to a medical specialist.

There are positives and negatives of exposing the emotional element within the debrief process; for some, it provides an opportunity for cathartic release to normalise what they have experienced, but for others the debrief process can open a wound that has not yet healed and lead to further trauma (Hawker et al., 2011).

**Benefits of debriefing**

Debriefing can change the culture of an organisation, by creating a relevant and timely discussion in a psychologically safe space, free from blame and judgement, enabling individuals to speak openly and safely (Copeland & Liska, 2016). The move from a blame culture is significant, and allowing individuals to speak openly creates an empowered work force that supports a learning culture which also seeks solutions. This empowerment is furthered when individuals see the outcome of the learning from the debrief being delivered.

For those who are part of a debrief process that utilises trained facilitators, the positive experience of being part of the debrief process is often an outcome recorded as good practice. This is furthered with the consideration that the debrief process should be completed for other incidents where appropriate. The opportunity to generate learning using reflective practice in the form of a debrief and the implementation of the learning assists in reducing the same or similar mistakes being made and provides opportunities for those on the front line to be involved in the solution.

For some, the first opportunity they have had to speak about the incident is during the debrief, and the ability to talk it through and rationalise thoughts and feelings can be hugely beneficial (Snowdon, 2021). Additionally, there are some tangible benefits of debriefing – for example, when debriefing a regular annual event or process, the debrief can create efficiency savings through better understanding of how a resource or function was used, which enables amended planning in the future. Debriefing can streamline current processes and procedures, reduce demands on frontline staff, and improve both team and individual performance by 20–25 per cent (Tannenbaum & Cerasoli, 2013). Anything can be debriefed, big or small, internal or external, and debriefing will uncover lessons (Swerdlow, 2018).

## Reasons not to debrief

There will be occasions when it is not appropriate to hold a debrief process, and organisations may need to take advice from legal departments to understand this.

If the incident is part of an ongoing criminal investigation, this alone does not prevent a debrief process happening, but it will guide the terms of reference for the debrief and what can be debriefed. Referencing some of the recent terror attacks, it was totally appropriate to debrief the initial response of those attending the scene to ensure the learning was captured and shared, but it would not have been appropriate to debrief the ongoing investigation due to the sensitivities associated with that.

If the rationale for holding a debrief is to identify blame, there should not be a debrief. Reviews and investigation processes exist if the organisation is looking for culpability; the debrief process should be free from individual blame and focus on organisational learning (Perri et al., 2021).

## Understanding the considerations/recommendations

Learning from incidents goes beyond simply identifying what went well or areas for improvement through the debrief process. This information is beneficial in determining responses to future events, but what needs to be acknowledged is that the debrief is not completed just to be part of a 'tickbox exercise' where the report is then filed and the learning not acted upon. Learning has only been truly achieved when a change is implemented as a result of the debrief (National Fire and Rescue Service, 2018).

The learning from a debrief process can be grouped into themes dependent on the organisation requesting the debrief; these include communication, policy and process, resources, equipment, command/management, and structure. Grouping the learning into areas can simplify the understanding of the debrief process (Simoni et al., 2019). The capture of good practice is just as important as recognising the areas for improvement, and it is important that this is discussed and recorded – understanding why something worked well is just as important as knowing why something did not work.

## Conclusion

Debriefing can be completed in a variety of forms and varies across organisations. The principles and the outcomes overall are very similar, and if achieved, the process is viewed positively. Debriefing should not be part of a checklist that is not progressed or that is used to identify blame; this will take organisations back to the blame culture that many have worked so hard to change.

To ensure the success of debriefing, organisations need to ensure it is part of a learning culture where recommendations and good practice are taken forward.

Investment in a facilitated debrief, involving trained facilitators, provides those being debriefed with confidence that the organisation is investing in the process. This is furthered if those involved can see that the findings are acted upon and positive change occurs.

## References

Allen, J. A., Reiter-Palmon, R., Crowe, J., & Scott, C. (2018). Debriefs: Teams learning from doing in context. *The American Psychologist*, 73(4), 504–516.

Charman, S. (2014). Blue light communities: Cultural interoperability and shared learning between ambulance staff and police officers in emergency response. *Policing & Society*, 24(1), 102–119.

Cheng, A., Eppich, W., Epps, C., Kolbe, M., Meguerdichian, M., & Grant V. (2021). Embracing informed learner self-assessment during debriefing: The art of plus-delta. *Advances in Simulation*, 6(1), 1–9.

College of Policing (2022a). Rapid debrief process – Essex Police. Available from: www.college.police.uk/homicide-prevention/rapid-debrief-process

College of Policing (2022b) APP (authorised professional practice) – Emergency Preparedness. Available from: www.college.police.uk/app

Colleen, R., Shannon, D., Patricia, C., Penny, H., & Tracey, S. (2021). Nursing and paramedicine student and academic perceptions of the two phase debrief model: A thematic analysis. *Nurse Education in Practice*, 51, 103001–103001.

Copeland, D., & Liska, H. (2016). Implementation of a post-code pause: Extending post-event debriefing to include silence. *Journal of Trauma Nursing*, 23(2), 58–64.

Dewey, J. (1916). *Democracy and Education*. New York, NY: The Free Press.

Edwards, J., Wexner, S., & Nichols, A. (2018). Debriefing for Clinical Learning. Available from: https://psnet.ahrq.gov/primer/debriefing-clinical-learning

Feuer, B. S. (2021). First responder peer support: An evidence-informed approach. *Journal of Police and Criminal Psychology*, 36(3), 365–371.

Firing, K., Owesen, V., & Moen, F. (2020). Organizational learning through debriefing: The process of sharing and hiding knowledge. *Scandinavian Journal of Military Studies*, 3(1), 169–182.

Gardner, R. (2013). Introduction to debriefing. *Seminars in Perinatology*, 37(3), 166–174.

Gibbs, G. (1988). *Learning by Doing: A Guide to Teaching and Learning Methods*. Oxford: Further Education Unit, Oxford Brookes University.

Gougoulis, A., Trawber, R., Hird, K., & Sweetman, G. (2020). 'Take 10 to talk about it': Use of a scripted, post-event debriefing tool in a neonatal intensive care unit. *Journal of Paediatrics and Child Health*, 56(7), 1134–1139.

Greenberg, N., Langston, V., & Jones, N. (2008). Trauma risk management (TRiM) in the UK Armed Forces. *BMJ Military Health*, 154(2), 124–127.

Grubb, A. R., Brown, S. J., Hall, P., & Bowen, E. (2021). From deployment to debriefing: Introducing the D.I.A.M.O.N.D. model of hostage and crisis negotiation. *Police Practice & Research*, 22(1), 953–977.

Hawker, D. M., Durkin, J., & Hawker, D. S. J. (2011). To debrief or not to debrief our heroes: That is the question. *Clinical Psychology and Psychotherapy*, 18(6), 453–463.

Hawkins, C. (2022) Debriefing, reflecting and being mindful are opportunities for us to engage in self-reflection. *Nursing Times*, 9 March. Available from: www.nursingtimes.net/students/debriefing-reflecting-and-being-mindful-allow-us-to-engage-in-self-reflection-09-03-2022

Healy, S., & Tyrell, M. (2013). Importance of debriefing following critical incidents. *Emergency Nurse*, 20(10), 32–37.

Hebles, M., Yániz-Alvarez-de-Eulate, C., & Villardón-Gallego, L. (2023). How to carry out organisational debriefing for team learning. *European Journal of Management and Business Economics*, 32(4), 436–451.

Kolb, D. A. (1984). *Experiential Learning: Experience as the Source of Learning and Development*. Englewood Cliffs, NJ: Prentice-Hall.

Kolbe, M., Eppich, W., Rudolph, J., Meguerdichian, M., Catena, H., Cripps, A., Grant, V., & Cheng, A. (2020). Managing psychological safety in debriefings: A dynamic balancing act. *BMJ Simulation & Technology Enhanced Learning*, 6(3), 164–171.

Kurt, S. (2020). Kolb's Experiential Learning Theory & Learning Styles. Educational Technology, 28 December. Available from: https://educationaltechnology.net/kolbs-experiential-learning-theory-learning-styles

National Fire and Rescue Service. (2018) *National Operational Learning: Good practice guide for fire and rescue services*. Fire Service College.

Neeley, M., Crook, T. W., & Gigante, J. (2023). This encounter isn't over yet: The importance of debriefing. *Pediatrics*, 152(3), e2023063198.

Omar, I., Hafez, A., Zaimis, T., Singhal, R., & Spencer, R. (2023). AVOIDable medical errors in invasive procedures: Facts on the ground – an NHS staff survey. *International Journal of Risk & Safety in Medicine*, 34(3), 189–206.

Perri, G. A., Lewin, W. H., & Khosravani, H. (2021). Team debriefs during the COVID-19 pandemic in long-term care homes: Essential elements. *Canadian Family Physician/Medecin de Famille Canadien*, 67(12), 908–910.

Scott, Z., O'Curry, S., & Mastroyannopoulou, K. (2022). The impact and experience of debriefing for clinical staff following traumatic events in clinical settings: A systematic review. *Journal of Traumatic Stress*, 35(1), 278–287.

Simoni, J. M., Beima-Sofie, K., Amico, K. R., Hosek, S. G., Johnson, M. O., & Mensch, B. S. (2019). Debrief reports to expedite the impact of qualitative research: Do they accurately capture data from in-depth interviews? *AIDS & Behavior*, 23(8), 2185–2190.

Snowdon, K. (2021). Exploring the clinical debrief: Benefits and barriers. *Journal of Paramedic Practice: The Clinical Monthly for Emergency Care Professionals*, 13(1), 1–7.

Sugarman, M., Graham, B., Langston, S., Nelmes, P., & Matthews, J. (2021). Implementation of the 'TAKE STOCK' Hot Debrief Tool in the ED: A quality improvement project. *Emergency Medicine Journal*, 38(8), 579–584.

Swerdflow, D. (2018) The Importance of Debrief and Reflecting. Idealist.org. Available from: www.idealist.org/en/careers/importance-debriefing-reflecting

Tannenbaum, S. I., & Cerasoli, C. P. (2013). Do team and individual debriefs enhance performance? A meta-analysis. *Human Factors*, 55(1), 231–245.

Walker, A., McGregor, L., Taylor, C., & Robinson, S. (2020). STOP5: A hot debrief model for resuscitation cases in the emergency department. *Clinical and Experimental Emergency Medicine*, 7(4), 259–266.

Zigmont, J. J., Kappus, L. J., & Sudikoff, S. N. (2011). The 3D model of debriefing: Defusing, discovering, and deepening. *Seminars in Perinatology*, 35(2), 52–58.

# 3 The theoretical and legal principles of formal investigations

*Jenny Shaw*

## Introduction

This chapter focuses on the theoretical and legal frameworks associated with investigations. It will provide an overview and summary of the main frameworks and legal considerations, identifying recent changes, specifically the new Patient Safety Incident Response Framework (PSIRF) introduced in August 2022. As the current direction in incident investigation argues for a move away from a root cause analysis (RCA) approach towards one centring on system improvements in the delivery of care and treatment, this chapter will align with that principle.

Theoretical principles for investigations provide a basis on which to conduct any examination of the circumstances of the incident, what factors to consider and address, and the identification of improvements to minimise the risks and recurrence of adverse events, and may inform and develop as the investigation progresses. Such approaches include human factors and **Systems Engineering Initiative for Patient Safety** (SEIPS) which are referenced in the SEIPS guidance (NHS England, 2022a) and are seen as key in developing a more collaborative, system-based response to learning from incidents and improving the delivery and quality of care and treatment.

The discussion around relevant legal frameworks includes a brief reference to areas to be considered, including the duty of candour legislation (Care Quality Commission, 2000) and the Health and Social Care Act (2014). This is dependent on the incident under review and may include the role of the police in certain contexts, such as mental health homicide investigations. It is important to remember that there may be specific legal issues which are to be reviewed and examined for individual cases. The areas highlighted in this chapter are, therefore, generic deliberations, and it is anticipated that investigators will make use of expertise and advice within their teams, services, and organisations to further appreciate any legal and practical issues.

## Theoretical frameworks

To appreciate the theoretical frameworks, it is important to remember that they do not, in themselves, outline 'how' to conduct investigations (such as methodology

DOI: 10.4324/9781003286240-5

adopted, including data analysis, interviews, and so on) but the overarching stance in interpreting and analysing the context and situational factors involved in an incident. Although the frameworks outlined are intended predominantly for use in healthcare settings (NHS and NHS-funded provision), they are beneficial to adopt in non-healthcare environments and settings.

The **root cause analysis** (RCA) (NHS Elect, 2023) framework has been used consistently in investigations in the health and social care arena. The main tenet of this approach involves identifying the main and underlying 'problem' which led to the incident (Uberoi et al., 2007). By asking repeatedly asking 'why' something happened at key stages (the 'five whys') and 'drilling' down to the main causal factor, the aim is to provide a linear explanation of the incident and to introduce actions and improvements to minimise the recurrence of a similar incident. Included in this framework is the importance of contributory factors, identified via a fishbone diagram or contributory factors framework. By examining the contributory factors, it is possible to identify those areas which may not directly align to causation, but which nevertheless provide an opportunity to improve specific care or service delivery arenas. However, there are limitations in the RCA approach – namely its ability to take into account the complexities of human actions and behaviour within a care and health context.

The **human factors and ergonomics** (HFE) model identifies the importance of examining where there may be failings within a system and where improvements can be made to avoid or minimise the occurrence of safety issues. This approach has been used in various sectors, including design, engineering, and aviation. Its adoption in the health and care sectors builds on the usefulness of the model in other areas and applies the principles to the activities involved in the care and treatment of individuals.

The main features or domains of human factors can be broadly divided into the following areas:

- The task or job, including the environment in which tasks are completed.
- The individual and their skills, personality, and understanding and acceptance of risk.
- The organisation or service, including its overarching culture, work practices, and leadership.

The exploration of human factors in health and care investigations aims to understand the wider context of incidents, considering why such events occur, from a more system-wide perspective (Holden et al., 2013). Analysis of the practices, culture, and individual characteristics associated with the completion of tasks offers a more detailed appreciation of the factors that contributed to the incident. In doing so, it aims to address improvements in practice that minimise the recurrence of incidents.

The **Systems Engineering Initiative for Patient Safety** (SEIPS) framework (Holden et al., 2013, Holden & Carayon, 2021; NHS England, 2022a) examines the relationships between work systems, processes, and outcomes, and builds on the principles of the HFE model. This approach has been given prominence in the new patient safety framework as outlined below, recognising the complexity involved in patient care and treatment.

As with the HFE approach, the model examines the following areas within a work system:

- **'Tools and technology'** – with reference, for example, to ease of use of any equipment, maintenance, etc.
- **'Tasks'** – this includes factors such as the intricacies relating to completing a work task.
- **'Organisation'** – namely, the working practices, pathways, and structures developed by the organisation, including policies/procedures and resource allocation.
- **'Person'** – including individual traits and team dynamics.
- **'External environment'** – this domain refers to those frameworks external to any organisation, such as regulatory and wider policy influences.
- **'Internal environment'** – this relates to the work environment and the conditions of this environment (e.g. lighting, heating, organisation of the physical workspace).

Through 'mapping' the factors and aspects involved in an incident, this model aims to provide an awareness of how they have impacted on working practices, identify those areas which were not effective or resulted in a negative outcome, and highlight key and achievable improvements.

Various tools are available to aid investigators in the utilisation of the framework and in understanding adverse events (as outlined in SEIPS 2.0 and SEIPS 101) (Holden et al., 2013, Holden & Carayon, 2021). As with the all the frameworks outlined, it is expected that those tasked with completing investigations will receive the appropriate training in order to undertake reviews effectively.

### The latest framework – Patient Safety Incident Response Framework (PSIRF)

Following the establishment of the Healthcare Safety Investigation Branch (HSIB) in April 2017, a consultation process began in March 2018 to examine the systems and processes for patient safety investigations. The consultation document recognised areas for revision and development. These included proposed principles for the revised serious incident framework: strategic, preventative, people focused, expertly led, and collaborative, as outlined in the NHS Patient Safety Strategy (NHS England, 2021).

In August 2022, the Patient Safety Incident Response Framework (PSIRF) was published. Alongside the new framework, supporting guidance and tools provided organisations and practitioners with a detailed guide as to the preparation steps needed for implementation, the key areas to introduce and the standards and principles to be adopted. An analysis of the framework recognises both the learning from the application of the previous framework but also the priorities of inclusion, collaboration, and system working. It is fundamentally a cultural shift, ensuring that the emphasis is now embedding improvement and learning from incidents in existing systems, plans, and actions.

### What are the main aspects of the new framework?

The standards accompanying the guidance give an indication of what areas organisations are required to incorporate and include in their approach to the management of patient safety incidents. It also removes the difference between serious incidents and patient safety incidents. The PSIRF requires organisations and practitioners to act 'proportionally' in response to incidents rather than adopting a prescriptive and narrow approach.

Under this framework, the use of data and the development of a 'patient safety profile' are advocated. This means that information is to be utilised to analyse in detail the factors and issues surrounding safety issues within a team, service, and organisation.

Four areas are highlighted to support the mobilisation and implementation of the PSIRF. As outlined in the framework guidance, these are:

1. **'Compassionate engagement and involvement of those affected by patient safety incidents'** (NHS England, 2022b: 4). This outlines the expectations that individuals, including the patient, their family/carers, and staff members, are involved in the process of investigating and learning from the incident.
2. **Application of a range of system-based approaches to learning from patient safety incidents'** (NHS England, 2022b: 5). As outlined in this chapter, the PSIRF asks organisations and services to adopt a systems-wide stance to incident management, involving active engagement with a variety of partners and stakeholders.
3. **'Considered and proportionate responses to patient safety incident'** (NHS England, 2022b: 5). This area refers to the application of proportionality, recognising the central role of improvement and learning. It also reiterates the removal of specific incident thresholds, asking organisations to identify case by case the appropriateness and opportunity for learning, whether through individual incident investigations or reviews or through the use of thematic analysis. This is further supported and outlined by detailed guidance.
4. **'Supportive oversight focused on strengthening response system functioning and improvement'** (NHS England, 2022b: 6). As previously highlighted, the PSIRF places improvement accountability – for example, the Integrated Care Boards (ICB) – as commissioning bodies in providing oversight and obtaining assurance as to the efficacy of the provider's incident management processes. Oversight incorporates specific roles and responsibilities across any system, and learning at the centre of patient safety incident investigations. This includes

effective and active partnership across the healthcare systems and is particularly evident in the area of governance. By governance, we mean both that internal to the organisation and the wider system.

As the new framework is currently being embedded in NHS and NHS-funded organisations, the practical application of its aims and ambitions is yet to be evaluated. As with any new policy guidance and initiative, it is anticipated that it will evolve and develop in accordance with key learning during its implementation.

## Legal considerations and principles

This is a complex area and involves several statutes (Acts of Parliament), law as determined in court cases (case law), and certain regulatory/mandated requirements for services registered, for example, under the Care Quality Commission (CQC). There are numerous pieces of legislation which may be applicable, dependent on specific characteristics. However, there are key areas that are relevant to investigations, including the accessing, obtaining, sharing, and disclosing of information during and after the investigation. Information governance (GDPR), confidentiality, and disclosure are defined by legislation and case law, which outlines the responsibilities and accountabilities for those dealing with information gathering, recording, and transferring. The regulations around the sharing of information between professionals, services, and organisations are particularly relevant in light of the emphasis on system collaboration, working, and improvement implementation in the new framework (PSIRF). Equally important are the requirements under the Duty of Candour regulation (Regulation 20) (CQC, 2000) and the need to actively engage and involve those involved in investigations and in improvement.

The table below provides an overview of legalisation, codes of practice, and relevant guidance.

Certain investigations will inevitably involve an awareness of other legal and regulatory processes and systems. This can range from individual disciplinary and professional conduct issues and responses, the requirements from a coronial law perspective (via the Coroners and Justice Act 2009) and those occasions where a criminal investigation is underway or in proceedings.

## Conclusion

This chapter has outlined, in brief, examples of the main theoretical and legal considerations and frameworks involved in serious incidents. Undertaking an investigation into such events can be complex and evoke a range of emotive and subjective perspectives, and should be seen within a wider context of national policy, specific directives, evidence-based practice, and regulatory requirements and oversight. However, in ensuring that a model or framework is adopted, it is hoped that investigations can achieve the overall aims of improvement, learning, and the reduction of risks in health and care environments and practices.

*Table 3.1* Examples of relevant legislation, codes of practice and guidance

| | |
|---|---|
| Information governance, information sharing and General Data Protection Regulation (GDPR) | Since May 2018, the GDPR sets out the legal framework for the management of data (including increased and explicit rights of data subjects) now enshrined in the Data Protection Act 2018. |
| Freedom of Information Act 2000 | This regulates access to information and disclosure of that information to interested parties. |
| Caldicott Principles and Guidance | This document identifies and outlines the eight principles to be applied when sharing patient-identifiable data. |
| Common law duty of confidentiality | This duty includes the requirement that information given in confidence must not be disclosed without consent unless for a justified reason (e.g. required by law or overriding public interest). |
| NHS Code of Confidentiality | This sets requirements for those working in the NHS and includes the need to:<br><br>• protect patient information<br>• inform patients how their information is used<br>• allow patients to decide whether their information is used<br>• improve ways to protect, inform, and provide choice. |
| Health and Social Care Information Centre Guide and Code of Practice on Confidential Information (2013 and 2014) | Guidance and code which outlines managing confidentiality in health and social care. |
| Records Management Code of Practice (2021) | This states how to maintain records in health and in care. |
| Duty of Candour – Health and Social Care Act 2008 (Regulated Activities) Regulations 2014, Regulation 20 | A statutory, regulatory (CQC), and legal duty to be open and honest with patients or their families when something 'goes wrong'. Various responsibilities are outlined, including providing an apology and an explanation as to what has occurred. |
| Human Rights Act 1998 | This includes reference to Article 2 (right to life) and Article 8 (the right to privacy for family life, home, and correspondence). |

## References

Care Quality Commission (CQC). (2000). Guidance: Duty of candour. Available from: www.gov.uk/government/publications/nhs-screening-programmes-duty-of-candour/duty-of-candour

Health & Social Care Act. (2014). Available from: www.legislation.gov.uk/ukdsi/2014/9780111117613/contents

Holden, R. J., Carayon, P., Gurses, A. P., Hoonakker, P., Schoofs Hundt, A., Ozok, A. A., & Rivera Rodriguez, A. J. (2013). SEIPS 2.0: A human factors framework for studying and improving the work of healthcare professionals and patients. *Ergonomics*, 56(11), 1669–1686.

Holden, R.J., & Carayon, P. (2021). SEIPS 101 and seven simple SEIPS tools. *BMJ Quality & Safety*, 30, 901–910.

Human Factors and Ergonomics Society (HFES). (2023). Available from: www.hfes.org

NHS Elect. (2023). Root cause analysis: Five whys. Available from: www.nhselect.nhs.uk/uploads/files/1/Root%20cause%20analysis%20%281%29%281%29.pdf

NHS England. (2021). The NHS Patient Safety Strategy. Available from: www.england.nhs.uk/patient-safety/the-nhs-patient-safety-strategy

NHS England. (2022a). SEIPS quick reference guide and work system explorer. Available from: www.england.nhs.uk/wp-content/uploads/2022/08/B1465-SEIPS-quick-reference-and-work-system-explorer-v1-FINAL.pdf

NHS England. (2022b). Patient Safety Incident Response Framework supporting guidance: Engaging and involving patients, families and staff following a patient safety incident. Available from: www.england.nhs.uk/patient-safety/patient-safety-insight/incident-response-framework/#engaging-patients

Uberoi, R. S., Swati, E., Gupta, U., & Sibal, A. (2007). Root cause analysis in healthcare. *Apollo Medicine*, 4(1), 72–75.

# 4    Family engagement – why it matters

*Julian Hendy*

On a bright Sunday morning in April 2007, my dad went out early to pay his paper bill. After talking to the newsagent for a few minutes, he was followed out of the shop by a man he'd never met or spoken to before – a complete stranger. The newsagent heard the man say, 'I know you.' Then, without any warning, the man produced a sharp kitchen knife and stabbed my dad once in the back and again in the neck, severing his carotid artery. They were significant injuries causing substantial and immediate blood loss.

Later, after his arrest, the man said he believed my dad was involved in a conspiracy with George Bush and the Prince of Wales to clone his children and give them sex changes to make them look like Kylie Minogue. We learned he had a lengthy, 20-year history of serious mental illness, drug abuse, and violence. He was known to carry knives and racially abuse his neighbours. The week before, his family were so worried about him that they asked for a Mental Health Act (1983) assessment, which, despite the reports of his increasingly psychotic behaviour, and even seeing large quantities of amphetamines in his possession, resulted in no effective action to keep him safe and well.

My dad died a week later as a direct result of his terrible injuries.

Nothing prepares you for this. My dad was fit and healthy, a kind and funny family man, much loved and well respected in the local community. Nothing prepares you for the knowledge that someone, however irrational, had deliberately set out that day to kill someone you love. I had so many questions. But the most important one was this: How could this have happened?

At the time, I'd been a documentary maker for over 20 years. I made investigative documentary films about terrorists, arms dealers, and war criminals. I'd been to combat zones in Bosnia during the Yugoslav civil war and was in Rwanda during the genocide. I'd even made films about people with schizophrenia in Brixton prison – some of the most tortured and desperate people I had ever met. I thought (probably naively) that with all this professional knowledge and experience, it would be relatively easy for me to find out the background and circumstances of

DOI: 10.4324/9781003286240-6

why the man who killed my dad was so unwell, so untreated and so dangerous that day. I couldn't have been more wrong.

I soon discovered that the NHS Mental Health Trust that had been looking after the man who killed my dad would likely be doing a serious incident investigation. So I called them to ask about it. Their first words took me aback: 'Who told you there's going to be an investigation?' Not 'I am so sorry for your loss' or anything even approaching that. (My mood wasn't improved when I later discovered that on the day after the fatal assault on my dad, the Mental Health Trust had sought out the perpetrator's family to tell them how sorry they were.)

I didn't realise it then, but it was the clearest demonstration of how health services can often just focus on the welfare and well-being of their patients and lose sight of the fact that there will be other people – family, friends, and others – who can be deeply affected by what happened and who are also in need of support.

It took me months to get a meeting with the Trust's medical director. She was a sympathetic woman, but she said she couldn't tell me much about what had happened in the lead-up to the attack on my dad. She said it was due to the offender's patient confidentiality; he would need to consent to the sharing of any information. I found this intolerable. They were saying my access to information about a very serious offence – the murder of my father – was in the hands of the very man who had caused it. That cannot be right.

## The national picture

It's more than 15 years now since my dad was killed, and in that time I've discovered that, unfortunately, my experience is not that unusual. Around 100–120 families are bereaved this way each and every year in the United Kingdom, a considerable proportion of the total number of homicides here. I established *Hundred Families*, a registered charity supporting families across the United Kingdom who have lost loved ones as a result of mental health-related homicides. It works with the NHS and others to improve services and learning, and to prevent further avoidable tragedies. Through *Making Families Count*, I've worked with hundreds of families affected by mental health-related homicides, families bereaved by suicide, and those with vulnerable children who have died in care.

I know very many families struggle to get information, assistance, and support from NHS trusts after serious incidents in care. Such information is often vital to help families understand what has happened and to assist them to begin to cope and recover from their terrible loss. I know as well that many trusts struggle to engage well with families, which has been documented, with depressing regularity, in many previous NHS investigations and reports as shown in Table 4.1.

Concern about this problem has led to increasing international academic attention and studies from the United States (Etchegaray et al., 2014, 2016) Canada (Vincent & Davis, 2012; Canadian Patient Safety Institute, 2017), Norway (Wiig et al., 2019), and the Netherlands (Bouwman et al., 2018) amongst others.

*Table 4.1* Previous investigations

| Investigation and year of publication | Investigation key findings |
| --- | --- |
| **The Francis Report: (Report of the Mid Staffordshire NHS Foundation Trust Public Inquiry, 2013)** (Francis, 2013) | 'The arrangements for public and patient involvement, and for local government scrutiny in Stafford, were a conspicuous failure.' (p.74) |
| **Independent review of deaths of people with a learning disability or mental health problem in contact with Southern Health NHS Foundation Trust** (NHS England, 2015a) | 'The involvement of families and carers in investigations of unexpected deaths has been very limited – 64% of investigations did not involve the family based on our review of the evidence.' (p.16) |
| **Report of the Morecambe Bay Investigation** (Kirkup, 2015) | 'Without the persistent efforts of some bereaved families, these events would not have come to light when they did … they raise understandable concerns about how widespread failures of this degree might be across the NHS.' (pp.184–185) |
| **The Report of the Gosport Independent Panel** (Jones, 2018) | 'Over the many years during which the families have sought answers to their legitimate questions and concerns, they have been repeatedly frustrated by senior figures … In the relationship with these powerful public bodies, the families have felt powerless. The Panel's Report gives voice to their historical concerns and substantiates them.' (pp. vii–viii) |
| **Learning, candour and accountability. A review of the way NHS trusts review and investigate the deaths of patients in England** (Care Quality Commission, 2016) | 'Families and carers told us they often have a poor experience of investigations and are not consistently treated with respect and sensitivity and honesty. This is despite many trusts stating that they value family involvement and have policies and procedures in place to support it … Families and carers told us they are frequently not listened to. In some cases, family and carer involvement is tokenistic and the views of families and carers are not given the same weight as that of clinical staff. The NHS underestimates the role that families and carers can play in helping to fully understand what happened to a patient. They offer a vital perspective because they see the whole pathway of care that their relative experienced.' (p.6) |

## What is family engagement?

The Healthcare Safety Investigation Branch (HSIB) defines family engagement as:

> The prompt, effective liaison between a family and an investigation to ensure the family is integral to the investigation and is treated professionally, respectfully and according to their individual needs.

(2020: 10)

It follows guidance developed by the police for specialist family liaison officers, deployed as part of the investigation following serious crime and particularly murder.

In Scotland, the Crown Office and Procurator Fiscal Service (COPFS) has described family liaison as:

> The process through which the Police and COPFS work together to provide victims and bereaved relatives with information and support during certain major investigations which may lead to criminal or other proceedings.
>
> (2021: 3)

## What does the current guidance say?

The Duty of Candour (CQC Regulation 20; Public Health England, 2020) requires openness, transparency, and candour after serious patient safety incidents. This means NHS provider organisations in England and Wales must do the following:

> Act in an open and transparent way with relevant persons in relation to care and treatment provided.
>
> (p.26)

> Tell the relevant person, face-to-face, that a notifiable safety incident has taken place.
>
> (p.19)

> Give 'reasonable support' to the relevant person, both in relation to the incident itself and when communicating with them about the incident.
>
> (p.20)

> Provide an account, which to the best of the registered person's knowledge is true, of all the facts the registered person knows about the incident as at the date of the notification.
>
> (p.26)

The 'relevant person' is defined as either the person who was harmed or someone acting lawfully on their behalf (Care Quality Commission, 2022). Previous guidance in relation to the investigation of serious incidents, the NHS Serious Incident Investigation Framework, said:

> The needs of those affected should be the primary concern of those involved in the response to and the investigation of serious incidents. The principles of openness and honesty as outlined in the NHS Being Open guidance and the NHS contractual Duty of Candour must be applied in discussions with those involved. This includes staff and patients, victims and perpetrators, and their families and carers.
>
> (NHS England, 2015b: 21)

The Serious Incident Framework was developed into a new Patient Safety Incident Response Framework (PSIRF) (NHS England and NHS Improvement, 2020). One of its main themes and principles is the promotion and support of 'open, honest and transparent' information with affected families. Patients' families and carers are considered active and supported participants in the process, and the Framework contains a section with guidance that specifically considers the meaningful engagement of families and carers, saying:

> Meeting people's needs not only helps alleviate the harm experienced, but also helps avoid compounding that harm. While we cannot change the fact that an incident has happened, it is always within our gift to compassionately engage with those affected, listen to, and answer their questions and try to meet their needs.

(p.5)

The General Medical Council (2019) also gives specific guidance for doctors:

> Following an unexpected death, there should be close adherence to the professional and statutory duty of candour to be open and honest with the family of the deceased. They need to be told as fully as possible what has happened, why it happened and be assured that they will be kept involved and informed throughout the investigation.

(p.28)

**What do families want?**

Our experience with families is that despite the complexities and singularities of each case, essentially, they want three things:

1. apology and accountability
2. recognition and respect
3. evidence of effective learning.

An apology often goes a long way when things have gone wrong. It's been claimed that some health workers consider an apology to be an admission of personal blame (and therefore to be avoided at all costs) rather than a sympathetic response to a devastating and serious incident. The NHS has even issued guidance on apologies 'Saying Sorry' (NHS Resolution, 2017) which confirms an apology is not an admission of legal liability, but the first step to learning and improving services to prevent further similar incidents, and always the right thing to do.

Families want to be recognised – a recognition that their loss is important and matters. In the absence of any communication, how can they know that health services know or care about what happened? All too often, we see that health services' primary focus on the patient can lead to neglect of their families, friends, and affected others, with a consequent failure to recognise their legitimate needs or offer any form of practical or emotional support.

We've also seen a routine distancing by health services from traumatic incidents. Patient deaths become 'untoward incidents'; cases where people have died become referred to by the Strategic Executive Information System (StEIS) number which facilitate the reporting and notification of Serious Incidents to relevant bodies. Real people are referred to by pseudonyms or false initials in investigation reports, robbing them not only of their names but also of their humanity. The failure to acknowledge and name the real person who has died – someone who lived and breathed, who was known and profoundly loved – can feel like a further insult and injury to many affected families. Many feel this could be so easily addressed with a little care and thought beforehand.

It's been well established that traumatic incidents can also have a devastating physical and emotional impact on those left behind. Evidence shows that it's common for them to become seriously unwell as a result, particularly with depression and/or post-traumatic stress disorder (Casey, 2011). Some people lose their jobs, some have to move home or take on new caring responsibilities in the aftermath, and some even turn to alcohol or street drugs in an attempt to cope. The failure to recognise and deal with this deep trauma arguably only stores up further serious health problems for the future.

Most of all, families want, wherever possible, for no other family to go through what they have had to experience – that if things have gone wrong, or could have been done better, effective and robust policies and practices will be put in place so the problems will not and cannot be repeated. Unfortunately, in our experience, this is where services often fall down. There have been countless 'serious incident' investigations and action plans, often coming to similar conclusions and repeating very similar recommendations. They just demonstrate that problems that have been previously identified and recognised are still occurring regularly and haven't been adequately addressed.

The Care Quality Commission's *Learning Candour and Accountability* (2016) report highlighted that there was often no consistent monitoring of serious incident investigations, along with insufficient challenge by governance bodies. They spoke as well of a lack of robust mechanisms to ensure action or disseminate learning. Similarly, *Mind the Implementation Gap* (Patient Safety Learning, 2022), a report on the continuation of avoidable harm following investigations after patient safety incidents highlighted four consistent themes within organisations:

1. An absence of a systemic and joined-up approach to safety.
2. Poor systems for sharing learning and acting on that learning.
3. Lack of system oversight, monitoring, and evaluation.
4. Unclear patient safety leadership.

Demonstrating and evidencing effective learning and improvement after serious incidents is the surest way of helping families and letting them know their loved one's death mattered and made a difference – that it had meaning and was not in vain.

## Some examples of what NOT to do: five case studies

### *1. Douglas Scott*

On 9 June 2007, Douglas Scott was fatally stabbed by his partner's son, a patient with paranoid schizophrenia. Mr Scott's family later met with the Mental Health Trust, which didn't go well. It went so badly that the subsequent NHS independent investigation (NHS London, 2011) felt compelled to make this recommendation:

> It is essential that East London and the City Foundation NHS Trust ensures that when serious untoward incidents occur … the person tasked with meeting with the family:
>
> - Knows the name of the service user.
> - Knows the name of the victim.
> - Is fully conversant with the care the service user received.
>
> (p.9)

### *2. Daniel Quelch*

Early on 23 August 2007, a patient of Sussex Partnership Trust broke into the house of Daniel Quelch, a complete stranger. He then repeatedly and fatally stabbed Daniel in front of his children (Hine, 2013). Senior executives of the Trust subsequently went to meet Daniel's family but were ill informed about what had happened. When the family told them exactly how he had died, the executives broke down weeping and were unable to continue, leaving Daniel's bereaved family to deal with the executives' distress.

### *3. Harry Morris*

On 18 June 2011, Harry Morris, a keen angler, took part in a fishing competition along the Sankey Canal in Warrington, when he was pushed in and held under until he drowned by a patient of 5 Boroughs Mental Health Trust. After many requests (and following the involvement of the local MP), the Trust eventually sent a copy of its Serious Incident Investigation (5 Boroughs Partnership NHS Foundation Trust, 2011) which was completely redacted for page after page and contained no useful information at all to assist the family to understand what had happened (Figure 4.1).

### *4. John Hall*

On 15 September 2013, John Hall was subjected to a ferocious and fatal attack by a patient of Northumberland Tyne & Wear NHS Foundation Trust. The assault (with a baseball bat) was reported to have left his face 'flattened and without structure'. The subsequent NHS independent investigation said: 'We reviewed all the

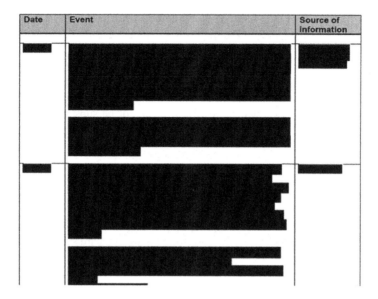

*Figure 4.1* Redacted notes

records and found no evidence that the trust made any effort to locate the victim's family so that they could involve and support them during the trust investigation' (Hyde-Bales & Jefferys, 2015).

### 5. *Elizabeth Thomas*

On 24 January 2014, 17-year-old Elizabeth Thomas was fatally stabbed by a former patient of Surrey & Borders Partnership NHS Foundation Trust, who was sectioned after the incident (Rooney, 2018). The victim's family were well aware of his mental health difficulties and were keen to know from the Trust if anything could have been done that might have prevented their daughter losing her life in such a terrible way. The Trust subsequently supported the perpetrator, his family, children at the school he attended, and the staff involved in his care. When asked about any support for the victim's family, the Trust said they didn't 'see a role in meeting the family'.

### Why is family engagement important?

Families can help improve the quality of serious incident investigations significantly, which, as discussed previously, has been recognised in the Patient Safety Incident Response Framework (PSIRF) (NHS England and NHS Improvement, 2020). They may have personal knowledge about key events and incidents that are not recorded anywhere in the medical records. They can help identify and fill in organisational blind spots and tell investigators what they don't know. This is evidenced by a number of different studies and policy guidance. The World Health Organization's Global Patient Safety Action Plan (2021) says:

> Patient engagement and empowerment is perhaps the most powerful tool to improve patient safety. Patients, families and other informal caregivers bring insights from their experiences of care that cannot be substituted or replicated by clinicians, managers or researchers. This is especially so for those who have suffered harm.
>
> (p.8)

The HSIB (2020) has written:

> Family members may be the only people with insight into what has occurred at every stage of a person's journey through the healthcare system. Not obtaining those insights results in an incomplete investigation.
>
> (p.12)

An academic study from Norway (Wiig et al., 2019) found:

> Inspectors considered next of kin as a key source of information that contributed to improve the quality of the investigation … Involvement of next of kin … contributes to a better understanding of work as done in clinical practice and contributes to strengthen the learning potential in resilience.
>
> (p.1707)

And another (Etchegaray et al., 2016):

> When an organization fails to ask patients and family members about factors contributing to their event, potentially valuable information from them is lost and not considered in the event analysis.
>
> (p.2601)

We have also found that the testimony of affected family members can often be a very powerful asset to help learning and improvement within health and social care services. Families' lived experience can bring home the reality of what has happened in a visceral way that routine medical records never can. Families' stories can be a very powerful aid to learning.

### Concerns and confidentiality

A common concern often heard from trusts is that they would like to engage with families more but are prevented from doing so by alleged 'patient confidentiality'. However, when questioned, health service managers either don't always appear to understand the existing NHS guidance and the limitations of confidentiality or otherwise immediately seek legal advice on why disclosure should not be made. Our experience is that health services rarely ask for legal advice on how they can best share information that might lead to a more open outcome.

In the cases we deal with – where people with serious mental illness commit very serious offences – we argue that the law is clear that there are limits to patient confidentiality and there is a balance to be struck between patient confidentiality and the families' right to know.

Lady Hale has said in the Supreme Court:

> There is a difference between cases where a court or tribunal is administering the property, care or treatment of a patient in his own best interests – and cases which are concerned with the proper management of a patient who has in the past been dangerous. There is a balance to be struck. The public has a right to know…
>
> (Hale, 2016)

In the case of Michael Stone, Mr Justice Davis considered the balance between Mr Stone's right to privacy and the family's right to information – that is, the balance between Article 8 (respect for private and family life) and Article 10 (freedom of expression) of the European Convention on Human Rights (1950). After very careful and detailed consideration, he determined that Mr Stone's right to privacy was reduced because:

> [the] justification for restricting Mr Stone's right to privacy [has] arisen out of Mr Stone's own acts – acts found to have been criminal. He has, as it were, put himself in the public domain by reason of those criminal acts, which inevitably created great publicity … Here the information sought to be disclosed relates – and relates solely – to the investigation foreseeably arising out of the very murders which he himself committed.
>
> (Davis, 2006: para 45.6)

Very few health services appear to be aware of this: that they do have solid grounds (and a legitimate defence) for sharing information with affected families after serious incidents. Sometimes it's claimed that health services cannot share information because they lack the expressed consent of the offender (who might refuse to share information or might be too unwell to have the capacity to consent), but again this lack of consent is not absolute.

Health services in England are supposed to have 'Caldicott guardians' to decide these questions. The are supposed to base their decision on certain 'Caldicott principles' including this one (Principle 7): 'The duty to share information can be as important as the duty to protect patient confidentiality' (National Data Guardian, 2020: 2).

Our experience is that some Caldicott guardians are either not well trained or have insufficient time and resources to consider the needs of affected families and fulfil the requirements of the role effectively.

## What are the risks of poor family engagement?

Poor family engagement can not only prolong trauma-affected families' experience, but it can also leave them stuck, not having the information to process what has happened and often leaving them alone imagining the worst (because if the necessary information is not forthcoming, there must be a reason it is being withheld, or the circumstances were so terrible that they have to be kept secret). Not knowing can be psychologically draining and poisonous, and can easily leave affected families angry, vocal, and upset.

The lack of effective and respectful engagement and a failure to answer legitimate questions can result in families feeling they have no other option but to involve members of parliament and the local and national media in prominent campaigns to try to get their concerns addressed (Buchanan, 2021; Townsend, 2021; ITV News, 2022). The failure to engage can also result in complaints to professional regulatory bodies, civil action, and enhanced scrutiny at coroner's inquests. All of these can lead to a widespread perception that all local services are poor and badly managed – a clear and substantial reputational risk to health services, which could be so easily avoided with better and effective family engagement.

Families who are treated well – with information, respect, and effective support – in general do not feel need the need to appeal to the media and wider public with their concerns.

## How can you improve family engagement?

We have worked locally, regionally, and with the devolved governments throughout the United Kingdom after serious incidents in mental health services and have developed the following principles to improve family engagement, which we suggest would form the basis of good practice.

### *Ten principles of good practice in family engagement*

1. Affected families will be identified and contacted as early as possible, and will be informed (and kept informed), of any investigation or review, if they so wish.
2. Affected families will be treated with respect and decency.
3. Families will be treated with openness and transparency and will be provided with the information they need.
4. The families' experience is important. They can add significant value and information that may not appear in official records.
5. Affected families will be supported to participate in any review.
6. Reviewers and investigators will be well informed about the case before speaking to families.
7. Communications with families will be clear and jargon free. (And there will be checks on the families' ability to read and understand English.)
8. Families will have a reliable, dedicated contact for any review process.

9. Families will be able to review and check the draft report in full for factual accuracy and will be given sufficient time to do so.
10. Families will know whom to contact, and have their concerns addressed by accountable services, if any of these principles are not met.

## Conclusion

Good family engagement not only helps affected families by answering their questions, treating them with respect, and recognising their loss; it also helps health services conduct better investigations, learn from what happened, and put effective measures in place to prevent further similar incidents in the future. It can help prevent further avoidable trauma, a drain on services, and a loss of public confidence in the safety of services.

Most important of all, good family engagement is what any family should expect when something terrible has happened to their loved ones. It is the right thing to do.

## References

5 Boroughs Partnership NHS Foundation Trust. (2011). Internal Review of Serious Incident. Available from: www.hundredfamilies.org/wp/wp-content/uploads/2019/12/OGBURN-Int-Inv-Jun-11.pdf

Bouwman, R., de Graaff, B., De Beurs, D., de Bovenkamp, H., Leistkow, I., & Friele, R. (2018). Involving patients and families in the analysis of suicides, suicide attempts, and other sentinel events in mental healthcare: A qualitative study in the Netherlands. *International Journal of Environmental Research and Public Health*; 15(6), 1104.

Buchanan, M. (2021). Southern Health: Bereaved families 'gaslighted and bullied' by NHS. BBC News, 29 January. Available from: www.bbc.co.uk/news/uk-england-hampshire-55856820

Canadian Patient Safety Institute. (2017). *Engaging patients in patient safety – a Canadian guide*. Available from: www.patientsafetyinstitute.ca/en/toolsResources/Patient-Engagement-in-Patient-Safety-Guide/Documents/Engaging%20Patients%20in%20Patient%20Safety.pdf

Care Quality Commission. (2016). *Learning, candour and accountability: A review of the way NHS trusts review and investigate the deaths of patients in England*. Available from: www.cqc.org.uk/sites/default/files/20161213-learning-candour-accountability-full-report.pdf

Care Quality Commission. (2022). What you must do when you discover a notifiable safety incident (duty of candour). Available from: www.cqc.org.uk/guidance-providers/all-services/duty-candour-what-you-must-do

Casey, L. (2011). Review into the needs of Families Bereaved by Homicide. Available from: https://samm.org.uk/wp-content/uploads/2021/01/Review-needs-of-families-bereaved-by-homicide.pdf

Council of Europe. (1950). *European Convention for the Protection of Human Rights and Fundamental Freedoms, as amended by Protocols Nos. 11 and 14*, 4 November 1950, ETS 5. Available from: www.refworld.org/docid/3ae6b3b04.html

Crown Office and Prosecutor Fiscal Service. (2021). Family Liaison: Joint working with ACPOS and COPFS. Available from: www.copfs.gov.uk/publications/family-liaison-joint-working-with-acpos-and-copfs

Davis, Mr Justice. (2006). *Michael Stone v Southeast Coast Strategic Health Authority* [2006] EWHC 1668. Available from: www.bailii.org/ew/cases/EWHC/Admin/2006/1668.html

Etchegaray, J. M., Ottosen, M. J., Aigbe, A., Sedlock, E., Sage, W. M., Bell, S. K., Gallagher, T. H., & Thomas, E. J. (2016). Patients as partners in learning from unexpected events. *Health Service Research*, 51(Suppl 3), 2600–2614.

Etchegaray, J. M., Ottosen, M. J., Burress, L., Sage, W. M., Bell, S. K., Gallagher, T. H., & Thomas, E. J. (2014). Structuring patient and family involvement in medical error event disclosure and analysis. *Health Affairs*, 33, 46–52.

Francis, R. (2013). *Report of the Mid Staffordshire NHS Trust Public Inquiry – Executive Summary*. London: The Stationery Office.

General Medical Council. (2019). *Independent review of gross negligence manslaughter and culpable homicide*. Available from: www.gmc-uk.org/-/media/documents/independent-review-of-gross-negligence-manslaughter-and-culpable-homicide—final-report_pd-78716610.pdf

Hale, Lady. (2016). *R (on the application of C) (Appellant) v Secretary of State for Justice (Respondent)*. Available from: www.bailii.org/uk/cases/UKSC/2016/2.html

Healthcare Safety Investigation Branch. (2020). *National Learning Report. Giving families a voice: HSIB's approach to patient and family engagement during investigations*. Available from: www.hssib.org.uk/patient-safety-investigations/giving-families-a-voice/investigation-report

Hine, N. (2013). Schizophrenic Benjamin Frankum sentenced over Daniel Quelch manslaughter. *Maidenhead Advertiser*, 22 January. Available from: www.maidenhead-advertiser.co.uk/news/10191/Schizophrenic-Benjamin-Frankum-sentenced-over-Daniel.html

Hyde-Bales, K., & Jefferys, P. (2015). *Independent Investigation into the care and treatment of Mr B*. Available from: www.hundredfamilies.org/wp/wp-content/uploads/2016/06/NICHOLAS-ROUGHT-_-Sep13.pdf

ITV News (2022, 1 March). Grieving families launch fresh campaign for public inquiry into Tees Esk and Wear Valley NHS Trust. Available from: www.itv.com/news/tyne-tees/2022-03-01/grieving-families-want-inquiry-into-troubled-mental-health-trust

Jones, Rt Rev, J. (2018). *Gosport War Memorial Hospital: The Report of the Gosport Independent Panel*. Available from: www.gosportpanel.independent.gov.uk/media/documents/070618_CCS207_CCS03183220761_Gosport_Inquiry_Whole_Document.pdf

Kirkup, B. (2015). *The report of the Morecambe Bay Investigation*. Available from: https://assets.publishing.service.gov.uk/government/uploads/system/uploads/attachment_data/file/408480/47487_MBI_Accessible_v0.1.pdf

National Data Guardian (UK). (2020). *The Eight Caldicott Principles*. Available from: https://assets.publishing.service.gov.uk/government/uploads/system/uploads/attachment_data/file/942217/Eight_Caldicott_Principles_08.12.20.pdf

National Patient Safety Agency. (2009). *Being Open: Communicating patient safety incidents with patients, their families and carers*. Available from: www.hsj.co.uk/download?ac=1293677

NHS England. (2015a). *Independent review of deaths of people with a Learning Disability or Mental Health problem in contact with Southern Health NHS Foundation Trust April 2011 to March 2015*. Available from: www.england.nhs.uk/south/wp-content/uploads/sites/6/2015/12/mazars-rep.pdf

NHS England. (2015b). *Serious Incident Framework: Supporting learning to prevent recurrence.* Available from: www.england.nhs.uk/patientsafety/wp-content/uploads/sites/32/2015/04/serious-incidnt-framwrk-upd2.pdf

NHS England and NHS Improvement. (2020). *Patient Safety Incident Response Framework 2020.* Available from: www.england.nhs.uk/wp-content/uploads/2020/08/200312_Introductory_version_of_Patient_Safety_Incident_Response_Framework_FINAL.pdf

NHS London. (2011). *An independent investigation into the care and treatment of service user Mr SUA.* Available from: https://hundredfamilies.org/wp/wp-content/uploads/2013/12/Alexander_Quintana_LON_06.07.pdf

NHS Resolution. (2017). *Saying sorry.* Available from: https://resolution.nhs.uk/wp-content/uploads/2018/09/NHS-Resolution-Saying-Sorry.pdf

Patient Safety Learning. (2022). *Mind the implementation gap; The persistence of avoidable harm in the NHS.* Available from: https://s3-eu-west-1.amazonaws.com/ddme-psl/Mindtheimplementationgap_ThepersistenceofavoidableharmintheNHS_2022-04-07-121554_vhao.pdf

Public Health England. (2020). Guidance: Duty of Candour. Available from: www.gov.uk/government/publications/nhs-screening-programmes-duty-of-candour/duty-of-candour

Rooney, C. (2018). *An independent investigation into the care and treatment of a mental health service user (S) in Surrey.* Available from: www.hundredfamilies.org/wp/wp-content/uploads/2021/07/STEVEN-MILES-Jan-2014.pdf

Townsend, E. (2021). Mental health trust fined £1.5m over deaths of 11 patients including 'beautiful son' Matthew. *East Anglian Daily Times*, 17 June. Available from: www.eadt.co.uk/news/health/melanie-leahy-essex-mental-health-inquiry-8065538

Vincent, C., & Davis, R. (2012). Patients and families as safety experts. *Canadian Medical Association Journal*, 184(1), 15–16.

World Health Organization. (2021). *Global Patient Safety Action Plan 2021–2030: Towards eliminating avoidable harm in health care.* Available from: www.who.int/teams/integrated-health-services/patient-safety/policy/global-patient-safety-action-plan

Wiig, S., Haraldseid-Driftland, C., Tvete Zachrisen, R., Hannisdal, E., & Schibevaag, L. (2019). Next of kin involvement in regulatory investigations of adverse events that caused patient death: A process evaluation (Part I – the next of kin's perspective). *Journal of Patient Safety*, 17(8), e1707–e1712. Available from: https://journals.lww.com/journalpatientsafety/Fulltext/2021/12000/Next_of_Kin_Involvement_in_Regulatory.141.aspx

# PART 2
# Conducting the investigation

# 5   Planning investigations

*Kevin Wright and Tiff Sinclair*

When one first reflects on the importance of thorough preparation before undertaking the review of an adverse incident, one could take the words of inventor and founding father of the USA Benjamin Franklin as a starting point that captures the essence of this chapter: 'Fail to prepare ... prepare to fail.'

When preparing for the investigation, it is vital that it is conducted sensitively, acknowledging the potential impact on those participating, especially the reluctant or fearful participant. This chapter focusses on NHS processes as exemplars of established protocols and procedures.

## Terms of reference (ToR)

The chapter will draw on the National Standards for Patient Safety Investigation as a framework for determining the scope of the actual investigation. Equally, it is a requirement of the wider NHS to respond to the requirements of the NHS Patient Safety Strategy (NHS England, 2019) in establishing internal mechanisms for investigation of safety incidents through an ethos of the 'just culture', whereby the investigation will seek to understand the context of patient safety and the human interactions that may contribute to safe and unsafe practices. Dependent on the nature of the incident, the terms of reference may be drawn from an agreed template within the organisation (e.g. lower impact, more frequent occurrences) or agreed with the recipients of the report (e.g. the board or executive lead for patient safety). It is anticipated that these in turn emulate the template set out in the Patient Safety Incident Framework (NHS, 2022a). Determining our response to patient safety incidents is complex, and guidance is available through the NHS Patient Safety Team to inform the nature and purpose of an investigation. Ultimately, the ToR should be informed by the desired outcomes as advocated in the above policy documents, and ability to learn from and bring about positive changes. Whilst the investigation is often feared (Goodwin, 2018), a prevailing sense of a functioning 'blame culture' will hamper the process of inquiry and learning; therefore, the ToR must signal to

DOI: 10.4324/9781003286240-8

all participants that the aim is to learn, not apportion blame on individuals or teams. As a template, these ToR will likely include:

1. **Purpose of the investigation:** for example, to identify the actions of a clinical team prior to and during a specific incident.
2. **Membership and responsibilities of individual members:** consider the expertise of each member and their application of subject knowledge. Identifying suitable specialists can be facilitated by such policy initiatives as the National Patient Safety Syllabus (Academy of Medical Royal Colleges, 2022).
3. **Declaration of interests:** whilst the investigation team may consist of external, independent members, in the majority of cases it will actually consist of those employed or otherwise engaged with the NHS provider, and therefore careful consideration of potential threats to the integrity of both investigators and the eventual report should be acknowledged.
4. **Governance arrangements:** whilst the use of root cause analysis remains the preferred approach, there must be agreement as to the use of this approach and whether an alternative approach may be warranted, such as the Concise Incident Analysis (CIA) tool (Pham et al., 2016). Additional guidance is provided by the Patient Safety Incident Framework (NHS, 2022a).
5. **Engagement of witnesses and patient safety partners:** although this is part of the governance arrangements and guidance is included in the Patient Safety Incident Framework (NHS, 2022a), issues of confidentiality and cross-agency communication need to be considered and agreed in advance to ensure appropriate management of highly sensitive data. Of course, the contact itself may prove distressing to the relatives of a deceased patients, so a sensitive, cautious approach is required.
6. **Agreement for triggers of investigation suspension**: whilst it is likely that the involvement of, say, the police or coroner's office will have been identified immediately following the patient safety incident, consideration must be given to factors that could trigger a suspension of the inquiry, such as the police investigation or if investigators suspect internal disciplinary action or investigation by a professional body may ensue. A pause could be required to allow this to be addressed. It would be prudent to seek legal advice should the investigation run parallel to such external investigations to prevent possible compromise of evidence required for civil or criminal investigations. Fortunately, acts of deliberate harm in health care are rare and require immediate actions to ensure the safety of all whilst preserving evidence.
7. **Reporting and communications:** the investigation will conclude in the production of a written report (usually following an agreed template), written in an inclusive way to ensure that it is suitable for all who will have sight of it. The investigator needs to know what is required (e.g. if an executive summary is also required, if the report is for internal circulation or will be used to inform other interested parties, including a patient or patient's family). The communication strategy also needs to be agreed, such as periodic reporting or advisement of immediate remedial actions required to support safe patient care and onward reporting to professional and regulatory bodies.

**Expertise of investigators**

Essential to the success of these investigations into patient safety and near-miss incidents is the expertise of investigators, who play a crucial role in identifying root causes, system-wide factors, and corrective measures, and in preventing future incidents.

Central to the recommendations made within the NHS Patient Safety Strategy (NHS, 2019) is a need to create a systematic and independent process for investigating incidents at local level, as well as growing investigative capacity within NHS trusts supported by a nationally led investigative body responsible for shaping the skills and expertise required to conduct patient safety investigations to a consistent standard. The Patient Safety Incident Response Standards (NHS England, 2022b) have made attempts to redress its shortcomings by providing standards of training and competence from patient response investigation leads that could be summarised in the follow key themes:

*I. Knowledge of healthcare regulations and standards*

Investigators need to possess in-depth knowledge of healthcare regulations and standards, as they provide guidance for conducting investigations and evaluating the performance of healthcare organisations and employees. Familiarity with regulatory frameworks, including those of the professional regulatory bodies such as the Nursing and Midwifery Council and the General Medical Council, is required. By adhering to these guidelines, investigators can effectively assess if organisations and individuals are operating within established parameters and identify deviations that may lead to incidents.

*II. Proficiency in incident investigation techniques*

Good investigators should possess solid skills in incident investigation techniques. This includes knowledge of methodologies such as root cause analysis (RCA), the Systems Engineering Initiative for Patient Safety (SEIPS) model, and the use of comprehensive, concise and/or multi-incident analysis techniques (Queensland Health, 2023) to navigate the complex structures, processes, and relationships in healthcare that impact patient safety incidents (Weaver et al., 2021). RCA, for instance, enables investigators to identify the underlying factors that contributed to an incident, whilst SEIPS focuses on factors related to the individuals, tasks, tools/technology, internal/external environments, processes, and outcomes that influenced the incident and outcomes (Holden & Carayon, 2021). Mastery of these techniques equips investigators with the tools needed to analyse incidents comprehensively and identify potential system weaknesses. Training programmes such as the NHS Patient Safety Syllabus V2.1 (Academy of Medical Royal Colleges, 2022) provide a framework for training for professionals undertaking investigatory roles, with NHS England (2022a) response standards recommending two-day formal training to achieve this.

### III. Understanding of clinical practices

A comprehensive understanding of clinical settings and practices is vital for investigators to effectively determine causality and identify contributing factors in healthcare clinical incident investigations. Debate exists around the strengths and weaknesses of local investigation team versus an independent team (Tingle, 2015). Local investigations have the benefit of rapid response to an incident as well as greater familiarity with the systems, clinical environments, processes, and barriers; however, Tingle (2015) observed a distrust in internal NHS investigations and a belief in a lack of independence and/or quality of investigation. The NHS Patient Safety Strategy (NHS, 2019) advises that the investigation team should include (or at least have access to) specialist knowledge, which could negate concerns about lack of local knowledge by including local knowledge in the team. Wiig and Macrae (2018) make a strong case for independent multidisciplinary investigation teams, observing that local-level investigations usually only work and influence within their own organisation (sharp end), whereas independent teams can review and influence at a regulatory, systems, and national level (blunt end). By possessing clinical knowledge, investigators can engage in meaningful dialogues with healthcare professionals, which aids in developing a comprehensive understanding of the incident's context and facilitating accurate assessments.

### IV. Strong analytical and critical thinking skills

In order for investigators to objectively assess complex incidents, they require strong analytical and critical thinking skills. Clinical incidents can often include gathering large quantities of data to review and organise into an accurate timeline and primary as well as secondary contributory factors. The aim of analysis is to establish 'what, who, how, why, and what can we learn' from the incident (Vincent et al., 2000), using a suggested adaptation of the Australian Transport Safety Bureau (Grey et al., 2011) analysis framework of a preliminary review, to identify themes and patterns, risk analysis, and finally an analysis review (NHS England, 2022c). By employing these skills, investigators can evaluate data, identify patterns, and recognise the causal relationships between various factors. Furthermore, critical thinking allows investigators to challenge assumptions, consider multiple perspectives, and arrive at evidence-based conclusions. These skills are essential for identifying systemic issues and providing comprehensive recommendations for improvement.

### V. Effective communication and interpersonal skills

Good investigators need to possess excellent communication and interpersonal skills as they will be required to interface with a broad range of stakeholders during the investigation, report-writing, and investigation feedback process. They must be able to interview witnesses, elicit accurate information, and appropriately document their findings. Additionally, investigators need to effectively communicate their conclusions and recommendations to healthcare professionals, administrators, and other relevant parties (NHS, 2019). Clear and concise communication is crucial, as it ensures that the investigative process is transparent and that stakeholders understand the significance of the investigation's outcomes.

## Timetable of activity and agreeing reporting of outcomes

The ToR should explicitly stipulate the timeframe for completion and reporting back from a clinical investigation (NHS England, 2022b). The recommendations for patient safety incident response times are one to three months and no longer than six months (NHS England, 2022b). This best practice guidance appears reasonable as delayed responses to clinical incidents can damage the organisation and individuals involved, and have the potential to lose momentum or see changes to the investigative team over prolonged periods.

Furthermore, duty of candour (also see Chapter 3) principles and guidance on engaging and involving patients, families, and staff require that stakeholders in the investigation should be offered opportunity to input questions to be answered within the ToR (NHS England, 2022d). At this stage, all parties, including the patient safety investigation lead, should agree on the preferred method for reporting findings both at draft and final report stages. Whether the investigation simply seeks to provide a timeline of events, subjective evaluation of impact factors for the safety incident or actionable recommendations will be established within the specific questions outlined in the ToR and scope of the investigative team's expertise. Regardless of the intended conclusion of the report, consideration needs to be given to the emotional impact of the investigation process as well as the outcomes for those involved. This will be considered separately in this chapter.

## Drawing up witness interview schedule

The Patient Safety Incident Investigation (PSII) guidance produced by NHS England (2022c) outlines a basic framework for undertaking an investigation once the need to investigate has been established.

1. Identify team/learning response lead.
2. Commence engagement with those affected.
3. Agree ToR.
4. Gather information.
5. Build narrative (similar to chronology or timeline mapping).
6. Analysis.
7. Safety action development.
8. Report preparation.

The process of gathering information is not specified within this guidance and will in part be informed by the ToR, the incident under investigation as well as, potentially, the knowledge and experience of the investigative team (e.g. a possible need to interview someone with specialist knowledge on a process or device). A 'walkthrough analysis' may be an effective way of understanding clinical processes or activities under investigation and allow the learning response lead to contextualise clinical activities, environments, and processes central to the incident under review adopting a SEIPS model approach (NHS England, 2022e). The PSII guidance (NHS England, 2022c) does recognise the synthesised nature of the steps 4–8 in the potential need to revisit steps once new information emerges which may result in new interviews or a revised view of the narrative. Vincent et al. (2000) suggest that a review of case records is the starting place before any interviews are conducted in order to develop a preliminary chronology and inform an interview list, and perhaps inform the order in which interviews are conducted. This approach may help to frame the issue and the questions to be asked at interview; however, a criticism of this approach has been clearly summarised by Clarke (2005) in his evaluation of the PEACE model of interviewing which was developed for police interview but has been adopted in the Healthcare Safety Investigation Branch 'guidance on the planning and conducting of interviews as part of a patient safety incident learning response' (NHS England (HSIB), 2022). Clarke acknowledges a potential for premature closure of an investigation, confirmation bias and/or selective synthesis of convenient details in the planning and preparation phase of PEACE (also see Chapter 6), which could be influenced by an early chronology created by case records alone and lead to such outcomes. A more uninfluenced preliminary chronology may be achieved by at least including the interview of active participants in the incident for review or a written account on which to base future interview.

When deciding who should be interviewed, the level and type of involvement, the ToR, and the information already known will undoubtedly influence the learning response lead's interview plan of who and in what order they will met (NHS England (HSIB), 2022). Those with direct involvement are likely to be interviewed earlier on in the process than those who have indirect or subject matter commentary, particularly where a chronology of events is unclear or incomplete. The reality of investigation preparation is that access to individuals can be a significant indicator of which order the investigations may take, especially where absence and sickness might delay proceedings.

Sensitive planning and consideration of the impact of investigations on the professionals involved will be needed for potentially unwilling 'witnesses' who may be invited for interview. NHS England (2022d) guidance on engaging staff, patients, and carers suggests that clear and transparent communication of the ToR as well as the review processes, along with the opportunity to contribute to system improvement, all contribute to a culture of openness and cooperation in the investigation process. Although an individual cannot be compelled to cooperate with the investigation process, failure to do so may result in further action, particularly if the professional involved is a member of a regulatory body for whom there is a professional expectation to contribute. All employees should be offered the opportunity to attend with professional body representation, as well as being offered support post incident and through the investigation process. Compassionate framing of the process to support the individual's voice within the review of an incident and focus on learning at a wider system level are suggested to reduce fear of being blamed at an individual level (HSSIB, 2021).

**Managing expectations**

Inevitably, there may be both internal and external influences on the development of the ToR such as the emotional investment of the family members of a deceased patient, public awareness of the incident and subsequent public scrutiny, and the need of clinicians to be reassured, exonerated even, by the process. The investigation will be conducted within set, possibly narrow parameters set by national and local policy and legislation which do not necessarily address the concerns of all parties, especially if 'blame' is the desired outcome by aggrieved individuals. It must therefore be emphasised that the patient safety investigation is for the purpose of learning and prevention of recurrence; if individual actions warrant further investigation via employee or regulatory mechanisms, then their contribution should not be utilised for this purpose without their agreement (and possibly their staff association) (Pinto et al., 2012).

**Support for the patient safety investigation lead/investigating officer**

The primary investigation lead can sometimes find themselves in a lonely place, with a burden of responsibility to thoroughly explore the circumstances of the incident and create an insightful and informed report. This can be incredibly stressful, not least because of a historical blame culture (Iacobucci, 2019) and a pressure to reach a position of transparency which supports learning and facilitates open dialogue. This is no mean task and requires a scaffolding of support for the investigation lead and (if relevant) the investigating team. Additionally, it is understandable that witnesses may be distressed by recent events and anxious about the process of inquiry itself, and providing a statement can prove to be cathartic for those colleagues giving evidence. The Patient Safety Incident Framework (NHS, 2022a) appendix talks specifically about the need for sensitive and compassionate engagement of participants, and recognises that the ongoing duty of care we owe to patients and colleagues alike cannot be compromised or impaired by the investigatory process. The provision of support mechanisms separate to the investigation is a plausible solution to include after the investigation's conclusion and submission of the formal report. Finally, of equal importance is the support required by the investigators as such incidents can be traumatic; it should be recognised that the investigating staff may need a 'safe place' and continuing managerial as well as clinical supervision. For instance, the investigation of patient (including baby and child) deaths or significant harm as a result of care failures will expose the investigatory team to any number of potentially distressing scenarios with patients and relatives, as well as staff members hostile to what may be perceived as attribution of blame that might bring their professionalism into question. Ongoing supervision, support, and debriefing mechanisms can and should be considered (Goodwin, 2018).

**Conclusion**

The necessity of an investigation into an episode of care unequivocally communicates its importance to those who contribute to its development through their testimony and to those who receive the final report and may also be tasked with

communicating its conclusion to those most invested in its outcome, whether patient, family or colleague. This chapter has sought to prepare the investigator for
the inquiry itself by identifying important preparatory steps. It also seeks to provide support to the investigators in this often-onerous task. Standards such as those
identified within NHS England's Patient Safety Incident Response Framework and
supporting guidance (NHS England, 2022a) offer those tasked with conducting
such investigations (NHS or not) an essential framework for the conduct of investigations. Furthermore, the skill and tenacity of the investigator themselves will
ensure that that final report is both an accurate and objective account that addresses
concerns and enables learning.

**References**

Academy of Medical Royal Colleges (2022) *NHS Patient Safety Syllabus*. Available from:
www.hee.nhs.uk/sites/default/files/documents/NHS%20Patient%20Safety%20Syllabus.pdf
Clarke, C. (2005). *A national evaluation of PEACE investigative interviewing* (doctoral dis-
sertation, University of Portsmouth).
Holden, R.J., & Carayon, P. (2021). SEIPS 101 and seven simple SEIPS tools. *BMJ Quality
& Safety*, 30, 901–910.
Goodwin, D. (2018). Cultures of caring: Healthcare 'scandals', inquiries, and the remaking
of accountabilities. *Social Studies of Science*, 48(1), 101–124.
Grey, E., Klampfer, B., Read, G., & Doncaster, N. (2011). Learning from Accidents: Devel-
oping a Contributing Factors Framework (CFF) for the rail industry. Conference paper,
HFESA 47th Annual Conference.
Health Service Safety Investigations Body (HSSIB) (2021). *Investigation report: Support for staff following patient safety incidents.* Available from: www.hssib.org.uk/
patient-safety-investigations/support-for-staff-following-patient-safety-incidents/
investigation-report
Iacobucci, G. (2019). NHS will focus on investigating serious incidents with the best learning opportunities. *British Medical Journal*, 366, l4514.
NHS England (Healthcare Safety Investigation Branch). (2022). *Guidance on planning and conducting interviews as part of the patient safety incident learning response*. Available from:
www.gov.uk/government/publications/the-nhs-england-healthcare-safety-investigation-
branch-directions-2022
NHS England (2019) *The NHS Patient Safety Strategy*. Available from: www.england.nhs.
uk/patient-safety/the-nhs-patient-safety-strategy
NHS England (2022a) *Patient Safety Incident Repsonse Framework and supporting guidance*. Available from: www.england.nhs.uk/publication/patient-safety-incident-response-
framework-and-supporting-guidance
NHS England (2022b) *The Patient Safety Incident Response Standards*. Available from:
www.england.nhs.uk/wp-content/uploads/2022/08/B1465-PSII-overview-v1-FINAL.pdf
NHS England (2022c) *Patient Safety Incident Investigation.* Available from: www.england.
nhs.uk/wp-content/uploads/2022/08/B1465-PSII-overview-v1-FINAL.pdf
NHS England (2022d) *Engaging and involving patients, families and staff following a patient safety incident.* Available from: www.england.nhs.uk/wp-content/uploads/2022/08/
B1465-2.-Engaging-and-involving...-v1-FINAL.pdf
NHS England (2022e) *A brief guide to walkthrough analysis*. Available from: www.england.
nhs.uk/wp-content/uploads/2022/08/B1465-Walkthrough-analysis-v1.1-.pdf

Pham, J. C., Hoffman, C., Popescu, I., Ijagbemi, O. M., & Carson, K. A. (2016). A tool for the concise analysis of patient safety incidents. *The Joint Commission Journal on Quality and Patient Safety*, 42(1), 26-AP3.

Pinto, A., Faiz, O., & Vincent, C. (2012) Managing the aftereffects of serious patient safety incidents in the NHS: An online survey study. *British Medical Journal* 21(12), 10001–1008.

Queensland Health (2023) *Best practice guide to clinical incident management* (2nd ed.). Queensland Government.

Tingle, J. (2015) Investigating clinical incidents in the NGS: A future roadmap. *British Journal of Nursing*, 24(8), 462–463.

Vincent, C., Taylor-Adams, S., Chapman, E. J., Hewett, D., Prior, S., Strange, P., & Tizzard, A. (2000). How to investigate and analyse clinical incidents: Clinical risk unit and association of litigation and risk management protocol. *British Medical Journal*, 320(7237), 777–781.

Weaver, S., Stewart, K., & Kay, L. (2021) Systems-based investigation of patient safety incidents. *Future Health Care Journal*, 8(3), e593.

Wiig, S., & Macrae, C. (2018). Introducing national healthcare safety investigation bodies. *British Journal of Surgery*, 105(13), 1710–1712.

# 6   Individual investigative interviews

*Alison Elliott and Karen M. Wright*

In this chapter, we will consider what 'investigative interviewing' is, before detailing two established evidence-based approaches to investigatory interviews. These approaches have been used in a variety of different ways where information needs to be obtained (Campanelli et al., 2016) and are used internationally (Paulo et al., 2015; Stein & Memon, 2006). We present these approaches since they are tried and tested with a range of witnesses – children, adults, and elderly people (Verkampt & Ginet, 2009; Wright & Holliday, 2006), with a range of delays between the event and interview (i.e. minutes to months) (Larsson et al., 2002), and for a wide range of incidents, including serious incidents such as crime or traffic accidents, and more minor events such as a phone call (Campos & Alonso-Quecuty, 1999).

## What is investigative interviewing?

Investigative interviewing is an approach for questioning victims, witnesses, and suspects of crimes, and, in the health/social care arena, practitioners involved in serious incidents or complaints, which is non-coercive and aims to obtain a full and accurate account of the events under investigation (Milne & Rull, 1999; Mendez et al., 2021). To do this they must ask the right questions, which may include the following:

1. In your own words, what happened?
2. Where and when did this take place?
3. What did you personally witness?
4. Who else was present?
5. What was your response or what actions have you taken since the incident?

However good the questions, the quality of any investigation will only be as good as the ability of the interviewer to establish and maintain a rapport with the interviewee, and to conduct each interview with a consistent approach to ensure rigour and fairness. The interviewee will not disclose to a person they do not trust or believe will use their information with respect. One way to make a good connection with the interviewee is using 'conversation management' (Shepherd, 1993;

DOI: 10.4324/9781003286240-9

Shepherd & Griffiths, 2021), described as an ethical, reflective, open-minded approach which is experienced as a mindful, managed conversation. This approach, known as the PEACE model, requires interviewers to skilfully create a relationship, where the interpersonal dynamics are carefully managed within the conversations to engender a commitment to reciprocity. This is done by engaging in skilful response behaviours such as showing respect, empathy, supportiveness, positiveness, openness, a non-judgemental attitude, and equality. For investigators who have clinical backgrounds, this sound familiar since it resonates with the work of the psychologist Carl Rogers, one of founders the humanistic approach which identified empathy, congruence, and unconditional positive regard as conditions for therapy (Rogers, 1951). The interview process is therefore an 'across' rather than an 'up-down' relationship with the interviewee, to minimise any issues relating to perceived power as far as possible.

## The PEACE model

The acronym PEACE sets out a five-stage process in an easy-to-remember mnemonic which we will explain in further detail, with examples:

P – Prepare
E – Engage and explain
A – Account clarification and challenge
C – Closure
E – Evaluation

### *Prepare*

In this stage of the model, investigators are advised to take some time before the interview to consider and reflect on their own personal style and the interview location. It is suggested that the interviewer prepares the general questions that will be asked during the interview in advance, pre-planning their interview strategy and considering who needs to be present (e.g. a note-taker). An experienced interviewer will be able to anticipate the responses of the interviewee; hence, good preparation will enable them to stay in control.

### *Engage and explain*

In this stage, active listening assists the interviewer to establish and maintain a rapport, identify topics during the interview and therefore manage the conversation. For example, the reason for the interview should be explained at the beginning by making a clear statement such as:

- 'You are here because you were involved in ...'
- 'You are here because you witnessed ...'

The interviewer should then check the interviewee has understood the explanation.

The objectives of the interview should be made clear at the very start, so the interviewer needs to provide an outline of what is to come. For example, the interviewer may say, 'During this interview I will talk to you about [list objectives]', and then go on to explain, 'I will also ask you about anything else that may become relevant during the interview in order to properly establish the facts and issues.' Repeated 'checking in' with the interviewee to check understanding shows respect and a repeated reaffirming of the focus of the interview.

During this phase, it can be helpful to anticipate areas of contention/disagreement, by using strategies such as asking the interviewee where they would like to start, as often they would prefer to get difficult issues out of the way quickly, or looking for areas of agreement – 'Remind me what we agreed on last time.' It can also be helpful to give interviewees a sense of control over small elements of the interview (such as who sits where) as small perceptions of control can affect levels of engagement. Finally, small, insignificant self-disclosures can help to lower the emotional tone of interviews (e.g. 'I used to work here', 'I hate this coffee', etc.).

### Account clarification and challenge

During this stage of the interview, the interviewer should be aware of the interviewee's non-verbal behaviours in response to questions and allow the interviewee to pause so that they can search their memory, without interrupting. The interviewer encourages the interviewee to continue their account until it is complete by using active listening and simple prompts (i.e. 'What happened next?' 'Then what?' 'Really?').

Awareness of the different types of questions and when to use them will enable the detail to emerge. See Table 6.1 for examples.

### Closure

This stage of the interview should be planned and structured so that the interview does not end abruptly. Where there are two interviewers, the lead interviewer checks that the second interviewer has no further questions before closing the interview.

*Table 6.1* Question types

| Question type | Example |
| --- | --- |
| Open-ended | Tell me, describe, explain. |
| Specific (closed) | Who did that? What did she say? Where do they live? When did this happen? Which ward was this? |
| Forced choice | Was the room warm or cold? Did nurse x or nurse y administer the medication? |
| Multiple | Where did he come from, which direction was he going in, and where did he go? |
| Leading | You saw the incident, didn't you? |

The interviewer accurately summarises what the interviewee has said, taking account of any clarification that the interviewee wishes to make, then any questions the interviewee asks can be dealt with. At the end, it is important to acknowledge what has happened and provide a brief summary, which also aids clarification. For example:

> Thank you for your time this morning. Your account of [the incident] will help us to understand what occurred ... So, just to make sure that I have fully understood, you saw ... so you did ... and afterwards ...

The interviewer then brings the interview to a conclusion by preparing a witness statement, or describing what will happen with the notes, and interviewee's right of review of the notes. Finally, they explain to the interviewee what will happen next.

### Evaluation

In this final phase of the interview process, which does not include the interviewee, the interviewer evaluates the content of the interview, with a view to:

- determining whether any further action is necessary
- determining how the interviewee's account fits in with the rest of the investigation
- reflecting on the interviewer's performance, and how this may be improved.

Although this PEACE model has many positive aspects, more recent approaches to interviewing of both suspects and witnesses have used techniques rooted in psychological theory, to elicit much more information and to ensure that the information obtained is reliable. One such model is the cognitive interview.

## The cognitive interview

The cognitive interview is an internationally recognised interview technique, used by police forces in a variety of locations including UK, USA, Brazil, and Australia, and in field studies and research. Here, we will consider it in the context of investigating serious incidents. The cognitive interview has been found to enhance hypermnesia, hence increasing the total amount of information recalled (Odinot et al., 2013), and studies have repeatedly demonstrated that this technique can increase the amount of correct information recalled, whilst maintaining accuracy (Verkampt & Ginet, 2010; Campos & Alonso-Quecuty, 2008). The cognitive interview has also been found to be effective when used with a wide range of people, including children, adults, the elderly, and those with intellectual difficulties (Clarke et al., 2013).

When people witness any serious incident or crime, they frequently confuse what they actually saw with their stereotypical ideas about people's behaviour (see Chapter 1). The cognitive interview has been found to increase accurate recall, without decreasing the accuracy of the information reported (Memon et al., 2010), and is effective whether interviewees are familiar or unfamiliar with an event (Ginet et al., 2014), although studies suggest that if interviewees are familiar with an event, then they are likely to recall more detail, some of which may not be relevant to the investigation. It is suggested that the cognitive interview typically generates considerably more information (25–100%) than a conventional interview (Memon et al., 2010) such as that suggested by the PEACE model. It does, inevitably, require the interviewer to have such skills, and formal training is advised in order to develop these.

The cognitive interview was developed by Geiselman et al. (1984), using cognitive mnemonics to enhance memory, and the core elements of the cognitive interview are organised around three psychological processes (Fisher et al., 2010):

1. social dynamics
2. memory and cognition
3. communication.

The cognitive interview was further developed by Fisher and Geiselman (1992) and further stages added, these can be seen illustrated in the Enhanced Cognitive Interview, which is presented later.

### Mnemonic one – Report everything

The interviewer asks the interviewee to recall everything they can remember about the incident, whether it seems trivial or not; otherwise, the interviewee may withhold important information they consider as not being relevant, or may choose to recall only such information as they consider relevant to the investigation.

Our memories for any given event may overlap, and 'irrelevant' recall may activate 'relevant' recall (Tulving, 1991).

It is important that interviewers do not interrupt interviewees whilst they are recalling, and it is suggested that interviewers take notes, as these can be useful when applying the other stages of the interview.

### Mnemonic two – Mental reinstatement of context

The interviewer asks the interviewee to mentally recreate the incident, and their physiological, cognitive, and emotional states at the time of the event.

Studies suggest that memory retrieval is more effective when the context of the original event is recreated during recall. This can be achieved by asking interviewees to close their eyes, or to look at a blank space/wall in the interview room, and to think about different moments of the incident. Notes from the first stage can be used by the interviewer to help fully explore mental images with the interviewee. To facilitate context reinstatement, statements should be in the past tense (i.e. 'When you went to …').

It has also been suggested that it can be useful to get interviewees to sketch this stage, and then describe what they experienced. This allows for them to use their own contextual retrieval cues, and it is less time-consuming and free from interviewers' interference, as it is the interviewee who directs the task and not the interviewer – the interviewer could inadvertently lead the interviewee – based on other witness statements, etc.

### Mnemonic three – Change order

The interviewer asks the interviewee to recall the event backwards, or in a different chronological order, as this has the potential to reduce 'script-based' memory retrieval (when interviewees recall events based on how they usually happen, rather than what did happen).

Changing temporal order has been shown to have a beneficial effect on the recall of correct information, and is especially relevant for enhancing the recall of inconsistent details. With this technique, overlooked details might be remembered, and recall accuracy usually increases.

This stage can be helpful in lie detection, since lying can be a cognitively demanding task, which may be difficult to perform simultaneously with other demanding tasks such as describing the event in reverse order.

The interviewer asks the interviewee to put themselves in the place of someone else present and recall the event from that person's perspective. Alternatively, the interviewee is asked to adopt a different emotional perspective – so if they report that they were anxious or scared at the time of the incident, they should be asked to take on the relaxed perspective they had before the incident. This is related to the principle of *varied memory retrieval*: different mental paths/cues can lead to the same memory. Reported information usually increases during this stage, particularly peripheral information (e.g. about the behaviour of others present during the incident).

In addition to the mnemonics, additional probes can be helpful. Generally, three types of probes are helpful in ensuring that as much information as possible is obtained (Beatty et al., 1997):

- **Cognitive probes** centre on people's understanding of questions, the information they drew on when answering the question, and the time frame they considered when answering the question.
- **Confirmatory probes** check that the information given by the interviewee is thus far correct.
- **Expansive probes** are used to get additional details from the interviewee.

There is some evidence that repeating the cognitive interview several days later can yield new information – as much as 21 per pent previously unreported information (Odinot et al., 2013). It has also been suggested by some studies that when interviewees are telling the truth, their answers to unanticipated questions are significantly more detailed (Sooniste et al., 2015).

It is suggested that the cognitive interview should not be thought of as a 'recipe', with a fixed set of questions, but rather as a toolbox of techniques, only some of which will be used in any specific interview (Fisher et al., 2010); however, the

Enhanced Cognitive Interview (Fisher & Geiselman, 1992) contains additional procedures which will be further explained and include:

- rapport building
- transferring control of the interview to the interviewee
- witness-compatible questioning
- mental or guided imagery
- summary and closure.

### Rapport building

Rapport building is the establishment of an appropriate and positive relationship with the interviewee, as presented in the PEACE model above. The interviewer should introduce themselves and take some time to explain who they are and why the interviewee is being interviewed. The interviewer should explain fully what's going to happen during the interview and show signs of active listening (e.g. saying 'mm' or gesticulating as a way of transmitting understanding), using the interviewee's name as a way of personalising the interview. Starting the interview by asking simple questions can also enhance rapport, and the interviewer should be aware of their own non-verbal behaviour throughout the interview to maintain rapport – if they are perceived as agitated/anxious by the interviewee, this will have an adverse effect on both rapport and recall.

### Transferring control of the interview to the interviewee

This is achieved by making the interviewee aware that even though the interviewer is there to help if needed, most of the 'work' will be performed by the interviewee, as they are the person that has valuable and relevant information. The interviewer should make clear that the interviewee has control over the production of information, and therefore may stop whenever they want to, and that they can recount information in whatever order they feel appropriate; by doing this, the interviewer is making sure that the interviewee feels more comfortable to talk about an event/incident.

### Witness-compatible questioning

This stage is about asking the right questions at the right time. All the questions need to be compatible with the interviewee's memory retrieval pattern – for example, if an interviewee describing an incident refers to a patient entering the room, the interviewer shouldn't simultaneously ask questions about what happened when the patient left the room, or who else was present, as this would interfere with the interviewee's memory retrieval cues.[1] Therefore, the interviewer should always ask questions that are compatible with the information that the interviewee is describing at that moment.

The type of questions used is also important, as highlighted above (Table 6.1). For example, closed/forced-choice questions should be avoided because they limit the interviewee's response possibilities and can produce incorrect information. Also, if an interviewer asks an interviewee closed (or forced-choice) question such as 'Did they use a knife or broken bottle to stab the victim?', this implies that they already know a weapon was used, which may be inaccurate or misleading and may distort the interviewee's memory; it may also limit the interviewee's response possibilities. By contrast, open-ended questions – for example, 'Tell me more about what you saw' – elicit more information and are less suggestible. Questions in the negative form – for example, 'He didn't have a weapon, did he?' – and complex/multiple questions – for example, 'Describe the attacker's clothes, what he did after, who else was present, and the other people's reactions to what happened' – should be avoided as interviewees can become confused and misinterpret them.

### *Mental or guided imagery*

This is similar to the context reinstatement stage of the cognitive interview, but instead of asking the interviewee to recreate large-scale scenarios such as 'What was the ward like at the time of the incident?', the interviewer asks the interviewee to recreate more specific details by asking questions such as 'What was playing on the radio?', 'What was on the TV?', 'What was the patient wearing?' The use of several sensory modalities is helpful as they activate different memory retrieval cues, therefore increasing the amount of recalled information.

### *Summary and closure*

At this stage, the Enhanced Cognitive Interview is very similar to the PEACE model interview, in that the interviewer should close the interview by summarising their interpretation of what has been recalled and requesting clarification This can potentially increase report accuracy and the amount of recalled information, and as the interview closes, the interviewer should check the emotional state of the interviewee, offer appropriate support and reassurance, and thank them for their collaboration in the interview process. This may enhance the possibility of interviewees coming back should they remember further information.

It is important to note that the Enhanced (and original cognitive interviews) are not 'all or nothing' processes, and that the interviewer should choose the strategies most appropriate to each interview, as well as the best time to use them. In terms of how to use these approaches, Griffiths and Milne (2010), suggest the following structure for an interview:

- Greet and establish rapport.
- Explain the aims of the interview.
- Initiate a free report (using context reinstatement technique and open-ended questions).
- Questioning (using report everything and witness-compatible questioning).
- Varied and extensive retrieval (using different perspectives and temporal orders).
- Investigate important questions (now the interviewer can introduce topics, even if the interviewee didn't yet mention them, if they are crucial to the investigation).

***Summary***

- Closure.
- Evaluation (evaluating obtained information and interviewer's performance).
- The Enhanced Cognitive Interview uses specific psychological processes to enhance memory retrieval. When we memorise something, there are three main phases:

  - Encoding
  - Retention
  - Retrieval.

**Encoding** is the first step for creating a new memory, which occurs when we have initial contact with the information to later be recalled. We would usually describe this step by saying we are trying to memorise something. Encoding can be intentional – when we memorise a phone number for later use – but also incidental – when we see something such as a road accident; we may not deliberately try to memorise details but would later remember several details (e.g. if told that the driver of the car had been injured). Some people (e.g. bank employees) can be trained regarding what information they should pay attention to during a crime, but this would not apply to most people, who may therefore struggle to remember some details.

**Retention** is the time between 'encoding' and later trying to retrieve the information. The longer this phase is, the higher the probability of a person having difficulty recalling the information and for memory to be inaccurate. Therefore, in relation to investigations, this suggests that to obtain the maximum amount of information, anyone involved in a serious incident should be interviewed as soon as possible after the event or invited to record their recall of the event (i.e. in the form of a written statement).

**Retrieval** is the last stage of human memory, which occurs when we try to access an encoded and stored memory. However, what is retrieved doesn't always correspond to the encoded memories, as retrieved information is often only a small proportion of the encoded and stored information and can contain distortions. The stages/mnemonics of the cognitive interview are designed to reduce such problems, as they enable interviewees to use successful retrieval procedures that psychological research has found to be useful.

### Psychological theory and the Enhanced Cognitive Interview

In relation to enhancing memory, the Enhanced Cognitive Interview is supported by two theories in relation to human memory: the encoding specificity principle and the multicomponent view of memory trace. The encoding specificity principle (Tulving & Thompson, 1973) states that memory is context dependent: when the context of encoding is recreated at retrieval, the amount of elicited detail should increase. Therefore, the context reinstatement and mental imagery mnemonics are important parts of the Enhanced Cognitive Interview.

The multicomponent view of memory trace (Tulving, 1991) states that memory is a network of associations, and the amount of coded information in storage is usually much greater than people can recall. Therefore, a memory can be accessed and retrieved by using several different memory cues. By using the 'report everything', 'change order', and 'change perspective' mnemonics, the interviewer is guaranteeing that several retrieval cues are accessed and that the gap between encoded and retrieved information is reduced.

Both the cognitive interview and the Enhanced Cognitive Interview have been found in repeated studies to enhance both the amount and the accuracy of information recalled by interviewees, and as serious incidents can be very complex events, involving multiple witnesses and their different perspectives, the Enhanced Cognitive Interview can be particularly helpful when conducting investigatory interviews (Geiselman et al., 1984). Other studies have found that this investigatory interview approach can provide a protective factor against misleading post-incident information (e.g. if an interviewee were to discuss it with another witness, before or between interviews, their memory may be distorted). Therefore, by using several different memory retrieval cues and asking interviewees to tell the same story using different procedures and sensory modalities, the effect of misleading information can be reduced and investigation report accuracy increased (Holliday, 2003; Holliday & Albon, 2004).

Finally, and perhaps most importantly, it has also been shown that both the cognitive interview and Enhanced Cognitive Interview are perceived as appropriate interview approaches by interviewees, and that the perception of 'appropriateness' has a beneficial effect on their willingness to be interviewed, their engagement, and their levels of recall (Paulo et al., 2015).

## Conclusion

This chapter has presented two examples of well-researched, tried-and-tested models for conducting the investigative interview. Clearly, the context in which the interview occurs and the presentation of the interviewee will lead the interviewer to use sensitivity and discretion in terms of the conduct of the interview. These models both present a clear framework which can be adopted in a multitude of situations to create comprehensive accounts and statements.

## Note

1 The interviewer's responsibility is to ask questions that are, effectively, 'retrieval cues'. These are prompts to trigger memories and need to occur one at a time.

## References

Beatty, P., Schechter, S., & Whitaker, K. (1997). Variation in cognitive interviewer behavior – extent and consequences. In *Proceedings of the Section on Survey Research Methods, American Statistical Association* (pp.1064–1068). Available from: www.asasrms.org/Proceedings/y1997f.html

Campos, L., & Alonmso-Quecuty, M. (2008). Language crimes and the cognitive interview: Testing its efficacy in retrieving a conversational event. *Applied Cognitive Psychology*, 22, 1211–1227.

Campos, L., & Alonso-Quecuty, M. L. (1999). The cognitive interview: Much more than simply 'try again'. *Psychology, Crime & Law*, 5, 47–59.

Campanelli, P., Gray, M., Blake, M., & Hope, S. (2016). Cognitive interviewing as tool for enhancing the accuracy of the interpretation of quantitative findings. *Quality & Quantity* 50, 1021–1040.

Clarke, J., Prescott, K., & Milne, R. (2013). How effective is the cognitive interview when used with adults with intellectual disabilities specifically with conversation recall? *Journal of Applied Research in Intellectual Disabilities*, 26(6), 546–556.

Fisher, R., & Geiselman, R. (1992). *Memory-Enhancing Techniques for Investigative Interviewing: The Cognitive Interview.* Springfield IL: Charles C. Thomas.

Fisher, R., Ross, S., & Cahill, B. (2010). Interviewing witnesses and victims. In P. A. Granhag (ed.), *Forensic Psychology in Context; Nordic and International Approaches* (pp.56–74). Cullompton: Willan Publishing.

Geiselman, R., Fisher, R., Firstenberg, I., Hutton, L., Sullivan, S., Avetissian, I., & Prosk, A. (1984). Enhancement of eyewitness memory: An empirical evaluation of the cognitive interview. *Journal of Police and Science Administration*, 12, 74–80.

Ginet, M., Py, J., & Colomb, C. (2014). The differential effectiveness of the cognitive interview instructions for enhancing witnesses' memory of a familiar event. *Swiss Journal of Psychology*, 73(1), 25–34.

Griffiths, A., & Milne, B. (2010). The application of cognitive interview techniques as part of an investigation. In C. A. Ireland & M. J. Fisher (eds) *Consultancy and Advising in Forensic Practice: Empirical and Practical Guidelines*, pp. 69–90. Chichester: John Wiley and Sons.

Holliday, R. (2003). The effect of a prior cognitive interview on children's acceptance of misinformation. *Applied Cognitive Psychology*, 17, 443–457.

Holliday, R., & Albon, A. (2004). Minimising misinformation effects in young children with cognitive interview mnemonics. *Applied Cognitive Psychology*, 18, 263–281.

Larsson, A. S., Granhag, P. A., & Spjut, E. (2002). Children's recall and the cognitive interview: Do the positive effects hold over time? *Applied Cognitive Psychology*, 17, 203–214.

Memon, A., Meissner, C., & Fraser, J. (2010). The cognitive interview: A meta-analytic review and study space analysis of the past 25 years. *Psychology, Public Policy and Law*, 16, 340–372.

Mendez, J. E., Thomson, M., Bull, R., Fallon, M., Hinestroza Arenas, V., Namoradze, Z., & Tait, S. (2021). *Principles on effective interviewing for investigations and information gathering* [Special report of the United Nations Rapporteur].

Milne, R. and Bull, R. (1999). *Investigative Interviewing: Psychology and Practice.* Chichester: Wiley.

Odinot, G., Memon, A., La Rooy, D., & Millen, A. (2013). Are two interviews better than one? Eyewitness memory across repeated cognitive interviews. *Public Library of Science (PLoS)*, 8(10), 1–7.

Paulo, R., Albuquerque, P., Saraiva, M., & Bull, R. (2015). The Enhanced Cognitive Interview: Testing appropriateness perception, memory capacity and error estimate relation with report. *Quality. Applied Cognitive Psychology*, 29: 536–543.

Rogers, C. (1951). *Client-Centered Therapy: Its Current Practice, Implications and Theory.* London: Constable.

Shepherd, E. (1993). Aspects of Police Interviewing: Issues in Criminological and Legal Psychology. Leicester: British Psychological Society.

Shepherd, E., & Griffiths, A (2021). Investigative Interviewing: The Conversation Management Approach (3rd ed.). Oxford: Oxford Academic.

Sooniste, T., Granhag, P., Stromwall, L., & Vrij, A. (2015). Statements about true and false intentions: Using the cognitive interview to magnify the differences. *Scandinavian Journal of Psychology*, 56, 371–378.

Stein, L. M., & Memon, A. (2006). Testing the efficacy of the cognitive interview in a developing country. *Applied Cognitive Psychology*, 20, 597–605.

Tulving, E., & Thompson, D. (1973). Encoding specificity and retrieval processes in episodic memory. *Psychological Review*, 80, 352–373.

Tulving, E. (1991). Concepts of human memory. In L. Squire, N. Weinberger, G. Lynch, & J. McGaugh (eds). *Memory: Organisation and Locus of Change* (pp.3–32). New York, Oxford University Press.

Verkampt, F., & Ginet, M. (2009). Variations of the cognitive interview: Which one is the most effective in enhancing children's testimonies? *Applied Cognitive Psychology*, 24, 1279–1296.

Wright, A., & Holliday, R. (2006). Enhancing the recall of young, young–old and old–old adults with cognitive interviews. *Applied Cognitive Psychology*, 21, 19–43.

# 7 Managing interpersonal dynamics and issues with group interviews

*Sue Ellis*

## Introduction

In this chapter, we consider the challenges of conducting group investigative interviews and of managing the interpersonal dynamics that may occur. It is hoped that this will create understanding of some of the complexities and will facilitate reflection on your own work in this area. Some of the specific approaches to group interviews are considered as well as some of the interpersonal dynamics which may occur. The impact individual members have on the wider group, as well as the impact a group has on individual members is also discussed, and additionally in relation to the wider organisation.

The human element needs careful consideration during the investigative process, and especially within a group setting which could be members of a team and/ or multidisciplinary. Despite the vast amount of education and in-service preparation provided to prepare staff working within roles relating to the risk and vulnerability needs of any clients, investigating serious incidents is rarely included, except as specialist training. The reality is that, despite the obvious best endeavours, things will go wrong, and there needs to be open dialogue within training, reflective systems, and management structures to acknowledge this and prepare for such circumstances (Bion, 1998).

## The personal impact of an investigation

The primary task of an investigation is for organisations to take learning forward to help prevent other similar incidents taking place. How the process itself is conducted is a vital component in helping to make sense of an incident and support all people involved, be that the service user, staff directly involved, or the wider team and organisation. The propensity for organisational anxiety is indisputably strengthened where there exists a negative, blame-seeking, and litigation culture (Francis, 2013).

It is critical to hold an awareness that whoever is involved in a serious incident will have the potential to be individually and/or collectively impacted on a personal and professional level and at risk of experiencing or reliving trauma as a result. It is important to consider individual and collective uncertainty about what happened

DOI: 10.4324/9781003286240-10

and is happening in terms of the individual's personal and professional responsibility, ethical principles, and professional body requirements. This may generate a deep fear of potential consequences for the person's position within the organisation and their future. It is important to resolutely comprehend the power of these dynamics, which may include fear around the potential loss of their professional role, career, identity, respect and status, and possible loss of income.

It is important to engage with all people impacted at the earliest opportunity, offering a containing and reflective environment that encourages and creates a structure to promote understanding around the importance and purpose of an investigation, whilst maintaining a safe, informed, and supported collective to explore the facts and to formulate the circumstances surrounding the incident. For some, it would not be appropriate to attend a group interview, but where there is a collective experience of an event, rather than an individual one, a group discussion can enhance memory recall, enable recollections, and create clarity around details.

Having clear structures, policies, and procedures in place for all staff can help contain the inevitable emotional impact, distress, experience of trauma, self-doubt, and fear in any necessary investigation. The process can vary considerably within organisations and in terms of other external agencies, such as professional bodies. However, the importance lies in all staff having access to current national guidance and regional and local protocols.

Chapter 2 considers the process of debrief, a process that is also often conducted in groups. Hence, it could well be the same group of people gathered to take part in an investigatory group interview who engage in the debrief process together.

The NHS Duty of Candour regulations first introduced in 2014 (updated 2022; CQC, 2022), as discussed in Chapter 3, provide a framework whereby services follow a statutory duty to be open and honest with people who use services, and others involved when something goes wrong that may cause harm in some way. Despite this being in place for many years, there is still a misunderstanding that genuinely saying 'sorry' is in some way offering an admission of liability, with potential personal and professional impact on an individual or group of staff. In practice, it feels understandable to think that by apologising there is an admission of guilt and that someone will need to be held accountable. When staff are interviewed together, as a group, their duty of candour can facilitate openness and an honest reflection on what happened.

## Group interviews

We will now explore some of the complexities and impact of dynamics in the group interview process, particularly where the investigation is potentially traumatic for those involved.

Although the similarities between incident investigation and research are many, there are many differences, and these are particularly important when deciding whether to conduct an individual or group interview. The most important difference is that in a serious incident investigation, those being interviewed may fear that they might be implicated, blamed or have their professionalism challenged.

Hence, sensitivity is paramount as the interviewee may feel vulnerable. Sim and Waterfield (2019) suggest that group interviews (*focus groups* in research) present several challenges for those taking part due to the uncertainty of what others in the group might say, creating unpredictable interactions. It can also be difficult to assure the individual of confidentiality, since other members of the group may speak of the conversation to others, outside of the group. Additionally, if a person becomes upset, they may feel more vulnerable if they are within a group of work colleagues. Sim and Waterfield suggest that strategies to fully brief and debrief the interviewees are crucial.

Whilst it is true that group interviews may feel more supportive and protective in some ways, they remove privacy that an individual interview provides. Group interviewees may feel under pressure to perform and may feel judged or scrutinised by others in the group (Ransome 2013).

There have been many theories and models of groups and group dynamics, although these largely refer to the group's transition as they work together. Tuckman's (Tuckman et al., 1965) model and Tuckman and Jensen (1977) have made a significant contribution to organisation theory. Tuckman suggested that all groups go through four processes in terms of group formation. This model has limited application in a group that meets only once, as in an investigative group interview, but it is worth remembering that the members of a group gathered for an investigative meeting are unlikely to work together as a discreet group, but rather a collection of individuals. Nonetheless, they are there for a single task, and therefore might well be seen to demonstrate some of the phases identified in Table 7.1.

During times of normal service delivery, complexities can exist and struggles occur from an unconscious, ambivalent position that rarely impacts to a significant degree, and is an indication that during times of stress, role conflict, and uncertainty, the customary and familiar dynamics can change. Group members individually and

*Table 7.1* Group processes

| Process stage | Detail |
| --- | --- |
| Forming | There will be little clarity on what is required and what are the roles and requirements. This requires the group leader or facilitator to outline the purpose, objectives, and relational aspects of the task. Processes are often ignored or unclear, and often all group members may be 'anti-task', particularly in situations of uncertainty, and this can generate individual and group anxiety that can reduce a team's ability to reflect and think. |
| Storming | Group members attempt to understand where they fit in relation to other group members. The task may become clearer at this stage, but the ongoing uncertainty and anxiety are likely to remain. |
| Norming | The group begins to understand the task and their individual and collective roles and responsibilities. This stage requires strong leadership to support the healthy functioning of the group. |
| Performing | At this stage, the group becomes more self-supporting and self-reliant and requires reduced interventions for the leader or facilitator. |

*Table 7.2* Group positioning

| The expert | This is the person who considers that they are the authority and have the most valuable interjections to offer, together with a perception that they are superior to all other individuals, including the group leader or facilitator, and will attempt to dominate the discussions. |
|---|---|
| The aggressor (actual or passive) | The individual who overtly or covertly attempts to undermine the knowledge and expertise and does not tend to be on task. |
| The indifferent | Attends because they have to, with little effort to interject with voicing their opinions, observations, and reflections. |
| Side conversationalists | Disruptive by engaging or attempting to engage in side discussions, particularly damaging to the person who is trying to engage in the process. |
| The one-track-minded | Stubborn, single-minded, and not ready to accept or listen to others' opinions; closes any further exploration of the discussions. |
| The uncertain | Not sure why they are there and individually lacking in self-belief and self-esteem, they can miss adding valuable input into the discussions. They may have a great deal to offer but miss the momentum of the discussions. |
| The talkative | Enjoys being the centre of attention and in the spotlight; has a view on all content. |
| The quiet | Very attentive and too hesitant to share their potentially valuable insights; caution is required by the leader or facilitator to help support their contributions. |
| The complainer | Comments on others – their colleagues, the service leads, the wider organisation, the service users. |

collectively may draw on past experiences in their organisational structure and culture to hypothesise on the outcome of an investigation (Grant, 1999).

We consider some of the common behaviours that can transfer the usual relational to a more transactional positioning (Adams, 1963). Table 7.2 shows some of the common positions that individuals can take up or are assigned during times of heightened anxiety and stress.

## Nominal group technique (NGT)

The role of the interviewer is, in part, to ensure that everyone's feedback and perspectives are listened to, heard, and processed. One recognised method for making certain that this is successfully managed is the nominal group technique.

This technique utilises a process that allows for identifying the problem, gathering information, generating solutions, completing feedback, and summarising before any formal report writing. One of the key benefits in situations where emotions may be heightened is to address some of the individual and collective anxieties around investigating incidents (Maguire et al., 2022). It can help if some individuals are:

- more or less vocal than others, to allow for quiet reflection for people who prefer quietly thinking
- ambivalent or anxious about the incident and the investigation
- not established within the team – for example, new members, people who may have been temporarily attached to the team
- supported if controversial or potentially sensitive issues are discussed, or there are pre-existing known complex dynamics within the team
- responding in a manner that alerts the interviewer to suspected power imbalances, perhaps rooted in leadership and followship relational complexity amongst the team.

The procedure is characteristically divided into five broad sections:

1. **Introductions and explanations:** The interviewer introduces themselves and invites each member to do the same.
2. **Generation of thoughts and ideas in silence:** Each group member is given a pen and paper with a clear summary of the subject for discussion. This is completed in silence with no communication.
3. **Share ideas:** An invitation to share with the group members. There is no discussion of the ideas at this stage, but there is further encouragement for individuals to write down any additional thoughts.
4. **Group discussion:** The interviewer encourages the group to explore others' ideas without judgement or criticism, but rather to approach with curiosity. Nothing is discounted at this stage.
5. **Voting and ranking:** The group explores ranking any commonalities in order of prioritisation. A collective outcome or hypothesis is proposed. The interview is then concluded with a plan for any communications clearly articulated.

There are pros and cons of this technique. The cons are that the process can take an extended amount of time to manage each stage effectively. Ideally, only one subject is explored, although additional linked subjects may emerge during the sharing of ideas and discussions part of the process. Team dynamics can impact the openness and confidence for individuals to speak, requiring the interviewer to hold an awareness of potential issues.

The advantages of NGT are that the process allows for the collection of individual perspectives as well as group opinions to further inform the investigation. The process can help rebalance a team experiencing difficulties around complex relational group dynamics. It also allows for all individuals to be heard equally.

**Conclusion**

In conclusion, it is worth considering the various models of group interviews before 'diving in', as well as the complexities of individual and group dynamics that might emerge in such a situation. Both those taking part and those facilitating the group interview need to be well prepared (briefed) and debriefed. Training for all staff is crucial in preparing everyone for involvement in such investigations and is, on some levels, inevitable during people's careers.

The quality and outcomes of the interviews rely on the relational influences between interviewer and interviewee(s). As humans, we all experience uncertainty, inaccuracies, and memory errors on factual information and chronology, particularly where there is stress and anxiety. Interviewers can exercise some control over potential influences on these factors and increase the amount and value of the information interviewees provide and ultimately the analysis and conclusion of the investigations (Strauch, 2002).

## References

Adams, J. S. (1963). Toward an Understanding of Inequity. *Journal of Abnormal and Social Psychology*, 67, 422–436.

Bion, W. (1998). *Experiences in Groups: and Other Papers.* Abingdon: Routledge.

Care Quality Commission. (2022). Regulation 20: Duty of candour. Available from: www.cqc.org.uk/guidance-providers/regulations-enforcement/regulation-20-duty-candour#full-regulation

Francis, R. (2013). *Report of the Mid Staffordshire NHS Foundation Trust Public Inquiry.* Available from: www.gov.uk/government/publications/report-of-the-mid-staffordshire-nhs-foundation-trust-public-inquiry

Grant, J. (1999). The incapacitating effects of competence: A critique. *Advances in Health Science Education Theory and Practice*, 4(3), 271–277.

Maguire, T., Garvey, L., Ryan, J., Olasoji, M., & Willets, G. (2022). Using the Nominal Group Technique to determine a nursing framework for a forensic mental health service: A discussion paper. *International Journal of Mental Health Nursing* 31(4), 1030–1038.

Ransome, P. (2013). *Ethics and Values in Social Research*. Houndmills: Palgrave Macmillan.

Sim, J., & Waterfield, J. (2019). Focus group methodology: some ethical challenges. *Quality & Quantity*, 53(6), 3003–3022.

Strauch, B. (2002). *Investigating Human Error: Incidents, Accidents, and Complex Systems.* Abingdon: Routledge.

Tuckman, B., Tuckman, B. W., & Jensen, M. A. C. (1965). Developmental sequences in small groups. *Psychological Bulletin*, 63, 348–399.

Tuckman, B. W., & Jensen, M. C. (1977). Stages of small group development revisited. *Group and Organizational Studies*, 24(4), 419–427.

# 8 Processing, reviewing, and analysing material

*Karen M. Wright and Alison Elliott*

*We would like to acknowledge the support and influence of Natalie Hammond and Georgia Warne in the preparation of this chapter.*

In healthcare, learning from incidents is essential in order to improve patient experience through the development of quality-assured, effective care, (Sujan et al., 2017). Following the investigation of a serious incident, it is imperative that learning occurs to prevent reoccurrence and establish confidence in the service. This chapter focuses on how a team might understand what may have 'gone wrong' and maximise the things that have 'gone right', to understand what may have contributed to a healthcare-based patient safety incident. It focuses on activity that occurs *before* the report is complete.

## Introduction

Since 2015, NHS organisations have investigated incidents under the Serious Incident Framework (NHS, 2015), commonly referred to as 'SI'. The focus of the SI Framework sought to ensure robust systems were in place for reporting, investigating, and responding to incidents, so lessons could be learned and actions taken to prevent future harm. Root cause analysis (RCA) describes the methodology for undertaking SI investigations and is used to establish how and why an incident occurred, in an attempt to identify how it might be prevented from reoccurring (US Department of Veterans Affairs, 2015). The 'five whys' technique is one of the most widely taught approaches to RCA in healthcare and is recommended by the World Health Organization (WHO, 2011). However, these approaches have been criticised for creating linear narratives for the cause of an incident and not clearly recognising the interacting contributions to the incident (Wu et al., 2008; Card, 2017).

Compelling evidence from national reviews, patients, families, carers, staff, and an engagement programme in 2018 revealed that organisations struggled to deliver under the SI Framework (NHS England and NHS Improvement, 2019). This resulted in the Patient Safety Incident Response Framework (PSIRF) (NHS England and NHS Improvement, 2020) which has replaced the SI Framework and should be used in all NHS investigations. The principles underpinning the framework guide the required approach:

**A broader scope:** describing principles, systems, processes, skills and behaviours for incident management as part of a broader system approach,

DOI: 10.4324/9781003286240-11

providing and signposting guidance and support for preparing for and responding to patient safety incidents in a range of ways, moving away from a focus on current thresholds for 'Serious Incidents'.

**Transparency and support for those affected:** setting expectations for informing, involving and supporting patients, families, carers and staff affected by patient safety incidents.

**A risk-based approach:** we think that organisations should develop a patient safety incident review and investigation strategy to allow them to use a range of proportionate and effective learning responses to incidents. The proposal is to explore basing the selection of incidents for investigation on the opportunity they give for learning; and ensuring that providers allocate sufficient local resources to implement improvements that address investigation findings.

**Purpose:** reinforcing the purpose of patient safety investigation and insulating it against scope creep and inappropriate use, so that safety investigations are no longer asked to judge 'avoidability', predictability, liability, fitness to practise or cause of death.

**Governance and oversight:** taking a different approach to the oversight and assurance provided by commissioners, emphasising instead the role of provider boards and leaders in overseeing individual investigations.

**Terminology:** making references to 'systems-based patient safety investigation', not 'root cause analysis', to reflect the 'systems' approach to safety.

**Timeframes:** instead of applying a strict 60 working day deadline, adopting timeframes based on an investigation management plan that is agreed where possible with those affected, particularly patients, families and carers.

**Investigation standards and templates:** introducing national standards and standard report templates.

**Investigator time and expertise:** requiring investigations to be led by those with safety investigation training and expertise, and with dedicated time and resource to complete the work.

**Cross-setting investigation and regionally commissioned investigation:** to better reflect the patient experience, co-ordination of investigation across multiple settings will be supported. This will include clearer roles and responsibilities for NHS regional teams to support investigation of complex cross-system incidents where needed.

(NHS England and NHS Improvement, 2019, pp.23–24)

Organisations are directed to develop a Patient Safety Incident Response Plan (PSIRP) which sets out how they seek to learn from patient safety incidents and includes guidance as to how incidents should be responded to. The move away from a 'one size fits all' approach allows organisations to utilise a range of tools depending on the nature of the incident and the ability to learn from what happened.

A patient safety incident investigation (PSII) is the highest level of response an investigation can provide, and focuses on a systems analysis approach, with the rigorous identification of interconnected causal factors and systems issues (NHS England and NHS Improvement, 2020). PSIIs should use improvement science methodologies to determine how to improve and make changes in the most ef- fective way, by systematically examining methods and factors that best work to facilitate quality improvement (The Health Foundation, 2011). A PSII should also consider the human factors including the environmental, organisational, and job factors and individual characteristics that influence behaviour at work in a way which can affect safety (Health and Safety Executive, 2022a).

A PSII can take between three and six months to complete and should be fol- lowed by a thematic analysis of similar incidents or findings to strengthen the wider understanding of care and service delivery problems and strengths to formulate robust safety improvement plans (NHS England and NHS Improvement, 2020).

### *Processing the material*

Following a patient safety incident, a debrief should take place (see Chapter 2). This provides staff with an opportunity to reflect and ensure immediate safety ac- tions are put in place to prevent similar incidents occurring.

An incident report form is logged and should include initial accounts from staff members involved in the incident. Coupled with a brief chronology of events from the incident report and clinical records, a decision needs to be made as to the scope of the investigation. Early review of this information will allow for identification of questions to be answered as part of the investigation, and this will be included within the terms of reference. Under PSIRF, the scope would be determined based on the nature of the incident and the opportunities for learning.

The order in which evidence is obtained may be key to the investigation, and a procedure should be available for the team that commissions patient safety investi- gations and the lead investigator to provide guidance as to what should be obtained. Any paper records from the clinical team should be shared with the investigator at the earliest opportunity.

In addition, there may be some evidence that has time-sensitive request applica- tions. For example, CCTV may need to be requested immediately after the incident as it may not be accessible after a certain time. There may be issues related to the General Data Protection Regulation (GDPR) (European Union, 2016) which the investigators will need to overcome to obtain what is required.

In contrast, postmortem and toxicology reports would need to be requested ex- ternally from HM Coroner, and these may take several months to conclude. There may be some incidents where there is alternative information from which to draw conclusions, such as the circumstances of death and a police report, instead of waiting several months for toxicology results. On the other hand, having this in- formation may be vital to the investigation, and therefore it should be noted that this would take the investigators longer than expected where they require external evidence (Health and Safety Executive, 2022b).

Examples of evidence which may be collated following a patient safety incident include the following:

- the incident report form
- staff accounts of the incident
- patient/family account of the incident
- paper copies of records related to the patient or the environment they were in at the time or prior to the incident
- photographs of the scene in which the incident occurred, which does not breach the patient's dignity and respect
- log and photos of equipment used during the incident, such as CPR equipment
- electronic copies of records
- CCTV, or other footage available
- access card/fob logs
- machinery data
- staff training logs
- details of staff involved in the incident, including their contact details as these might be required by the investigators during the investigation
- site visit
- details of any investigations completed prior (safeguarding, complaints, etc.)
- incident report forms for events the patient was involved in prior to the incident under investigation
- identification of policies and procedures to refer to
- postmortem and toxicology reports
- other investigations related to the incident which might be completed externally, such as police, neighbouring organisations
- information-gathering sessions/interviews with staff.

At each point the evidence is collected, this should be logged. The PSIRF provides guidance that this should include the following:

- identifier
- evidence type
- description
- origin
- date received
- outstanding tasks associated with the evidence or the request to obtain.

The evidence collated will assist the investigator in piecing together a timeline of events which occurred prior to the patient incident. Some evidence will be used to triangulate events, whereas other evidence types may provide differing versions of events. The investigator will need to reference the evidence they have used, as some types will provide more concrete conclusions than others. As an example, an initial account from a staff member may provide an estimated time of events, which can be verified with the use of other accounts, machinery data, and footage gathered. This will assist in strengthening the chronology and recognise any care and service delivery problems or strengths.

### Reviewing the material

Once the initial evidence has been collected and logged, it can be collated into a chronology. Evidence may have been obtained that does not feature within the scope of the investigation, and this should be stored but may not warrant reference within the investigation report. A chronological approach is important to make sense of events, and to feed into the ultimate 'storytelling' that will be expected in the dissemination process. Although the term 'storytelling' might seem childlike or even fictitiously constructed, a well-informed storyteller can make sense of complicated and dynamic information, collated within a chronological framework to provide an insightful, understandable, and accessible account. Shropshire Community Health NHS Trust's toolkit *Using stories to improve Patient, Carer and Staff experiences and outcomes* provides an excellent guide as how to use storytelling as a vehicle for learning from patient and carer experiences.

In relation to gaps in knowledge from the information that has been gathered, there may be occasions where the terms of reference and the scope require review. For example, where information shows a patient had been in contact with teams within social care, and where there are opportunities for wider organisational learning, a multi-agency investigation may be required. This would involve other agencies providing their chronologies, evidence, and information to assist with the investigation and jointly determine findings and learning outcomes.

Furthermore, review of the evidence and formulation of the chronology may provide the investigator with insight that further evidence is required. The process of obtaining further evidence may occur several times during an investigation. This is commonly observed with information-gathering sessions/interviews with staff members. As an example, two staff members have been contacted to obtain their verbal account; staff member A engaged with the information-gathering session to provide their account and answer the investigators' questions of the. Following this, the investigators met with staff member B, who raised additional points not previously covered with staff member A. This led to further questions from the investigators, who arranged to meet again with staff member A to obtain clarity.

Supporting staff to be open about mistakes allows valuable lessons to be identified, and this is a key principle within patient safety investigations (NHS England and NHS Improvement, 2022). A just culture considers wider systemic issues where professionals operating the system are enabled to learn without fear of retribution; where they are not punished for their actions, omissions, or decisions based on experience and training, but only when there is evidence of gross negligence and misconduct (Department of Health and Social Care, 2018; NHS England and

NHS Improvement, 2020). Hence, when constructing the material for the report, it is vital that an objective and non-biased approach is adopted.

PSIRF principles encourage staff members involved in the patient's care to contribute to the investigation. Whilst evidence may provide the investigators with clarity on what happened, the reasons why and how this occurred may not always be evident within clinical records or other forms of physical evidence, and therefore gathering this from staff members through verbal accounts is necessary. This is what will provide insight into the systems-based approaches to healthcare teams when considering the contributory and mitigating factors (NHS Improvement, 2022).

## Analysing the material

An investigation may harvest a huge number of documents, which might include reports, interview transcripts, communications (such as emails), professional records, protocols, and minutes of meetings. Sifting through this can feel like an overwhelming task for the investigation team and lead investigator. Fortunately, the Patient Safety Incident Response Framework (PSIRF) provides a downloadable toolkit which includes system-based approaches and tools that have been informed by the framework (Systems Engineering Initiative for Patient Safety) (Holden et al., 2013; NHS England and NHS Improvement, 2020).

First, screen and filter the material you have collected and determine if it meets the aim of the investigation and the terms of reference; you need to be sure that you have covered all bases. There is likely to be a fair amount of erroneous material too, which may provide context, but does not provide answers.

## Thematic analysis

You will notice here that we have reverted to the language of research here. Investigators are, indeed, researchers. They research the events that contributed to the need for an investigation and rely upon witness accounts and professional statements using much the same methodologies utilised in research. Furthermore, the trustworthiness of the investigation relies upon the same principles as research – that is, reliability, validity, and objectivity.

Thematic analysis (TA) and content analysis are time-tested approaches to identifying the meaningful themes that emerge from written data such as interview transcripts and statements. Joffe and Yardley (2004) discuss both in detail and provide pragmatic guidance for the coding of the data to identify the emergent themes. A robust approach that does not rely upon the opinion of one person but is also scrutinised by further review is recommended. Moreover, Clarke and Braun's (2021) approach to thematic analysis has become common parlance in qualitative research since it is the most widely cited of all approaches to TA available.

The PSIF advises that a table is constructed to highlight the barriers and facilitators, hence identifying what supports and what hinders work. It also suggests that an interactive map is constructed that enables a whole-system perspective to be displayed. This is further described by Holden and Carayon (2021) who also refer to this as the 'configural diagram' to show how systems and people interact to explain why something has happened and offer insight into consequential factors and interactions. They also provide a practice-oriented System Engineering

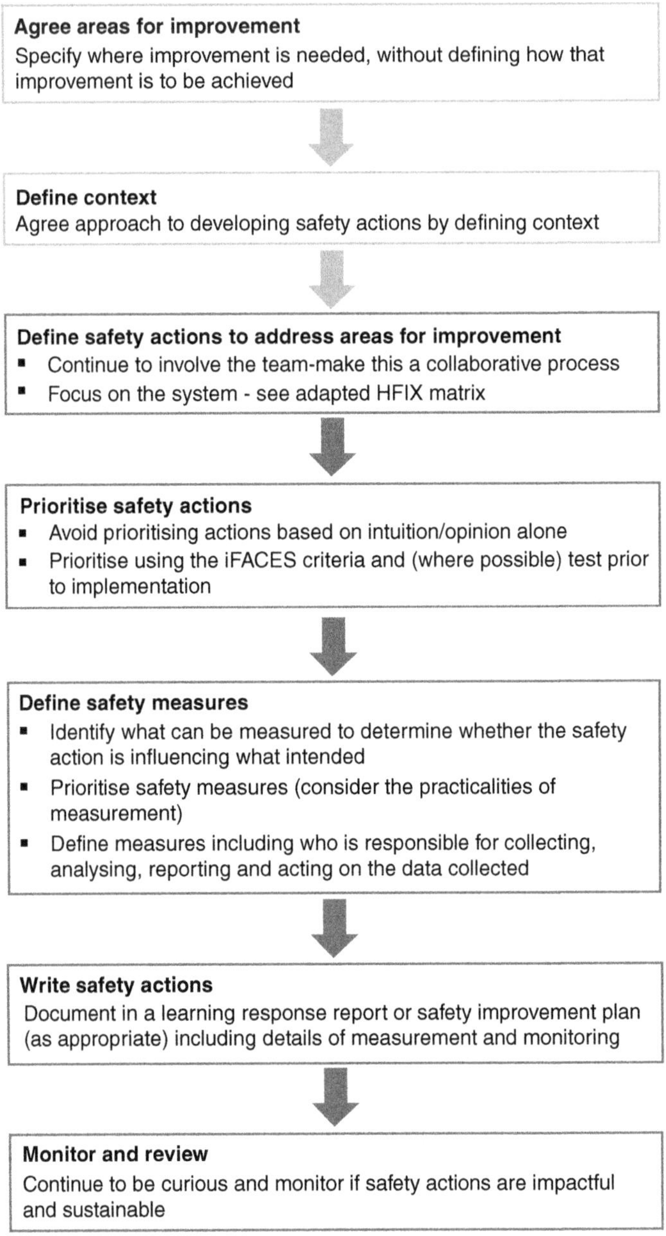

**Agree areas for improvement**
Specify where improvement is needed, without defining how that improvement is to be achieved

**Define context**
Agree approach to developing safety actions by defining context

**Define safety actions to address areas for improvement**
- Continue to involve the team-make this a collaborative process
- Focus on the system - see adapted HFIX matrix

**Prioritise safety actions**
- Avoid prioritising actions based on intuition/opinion alone
- Prioritise using the iFACES criteria and (where possible) test prior to implementation

**Define safety measures**
- Identify what can be measured to determine whether the safety action is influencing what intended
- Prioritise safety measures (consider the practicalities of measurement)
- Define measures including who is responsible for collecting, analysing, reporting and acting on the data collected

**Write safety actions**
Document in a learning response report or safety improvement plan (as appropriate) including details of measurement and monitoring

**Monitor and review**
Continue to be curious and monitor if safety actions are impactful and sustainable

*Figure 8.1* Overview of safety action development process
(NHS England 2022b: 6)

Imitative for Patient Safety (SEIPS) model which is broken down into seven steps (Holden & Carayon, 2021). SEIPS is a framework that provides a mechanism for understanding outcomes within complex socio-technical systems (NHS England, 2022a). NHS England (2022a: 1) identify healthcare as a 'a complex socio-technical system' due to its highly variable, uncertain, and dynamic nature, both technological and human.

## Conclusion

It is quite apparent that the investigatory activity, prior to the writing of the report itself, is an extensive process. Things don't simply 'go wrong', and an in-depth inquiry into the context of the incident, the people involved and human and organisational factors are required to enable us to gain insight into the contributory factors and the interaction between them. Fortunately, the NHS has provided a comprehensive framework which has been described here. Furthermore, the principles applied are largely transferrable to many other organisations.

## References

Clarke, V., & Braun, V. (2021). Thematic analysis: A practical guide. *Thematic Analysis*, 1–100.

Card, A. J. (2017). The problem with the '5 whys'. *BMJ Quality and Safety*, 26, 671–677.

Department of Health and Social Care. (2018). *Gross Negligence Manslaughter in Healthcare*. Available from: https://assets.publishing.service.gov.uk/media/5b2a3634 ed915d2cc8317662/Williams_Report.pdf

European Union. (2016). *EU General Data Protection Regulation* (GDPR): Regulation (EU) 2016/679 of the European Parliament and of the Council of 27 April 2016 on the protection of natural persons with regard to the processing of personal data and on the free movement of such data, and repealing Directive 95/46/EC. European Parliament.

Health and Safety Executive. (2022). *Introduction to human factors*. Available from: www.hse.gov.uk/humanfactors/introduction.htm

Health and Safety Executive. (2022a). *Evidence that may assist your investigation*. Available from: www.hse.gov.uk/enforce/enforcementguide/investigation/physical-evidence.htm

Holden, R. J., & Carayon, P. (2021). SEIPS 101 and seven simple SEIPS tools. *BMJ Quality & Safety*, 30(11), 901–910.

Holden, R. J., Carayon, P., Gurses, A. P., Hoonakker, P., Hundt, A. S., Ozok, A. A., & Rivera-Rodriguez, A. J. (2013). SEIPS 2.0: A human factors framework for studying and improving the work of healthcare professionals and patients. *Ergonomics*, 56(11), 1669–1686.

Joffe, H., & Yardley, L. (2004). *Content and Thematic Analysis. Research Methods for Clinical and Health Psychology* (pp.56–68). London: Sage.

NHS England. (2015). *Serious Incident Framework*. Available from: www.england.nhs.uk/patient-safety/serious-incident-framework

NHS England and NHS Improvement. (2019). *The NHS Patient Safety Strategy: Safer culture, safer systems, safer patients*. Available from: www.england.nhs.uk/wp-content/uploads/2020/08/190708_Patient_Safety_Strategy_for_website_v4.pdf

NHS England and NHS Improvement. (2020). *National standards for patient safety investigation.* Available from: www.england.nhs.uk/patient-safety/patient-safety-improvement-programme

NHS England and NHS Improvement. (2022). *A just culture guide.* Available from: www.england.nhs.uk/wp-content/uploads/2021/02/NHS_0932_JC_Poster_A3.pdf

NHS England. (2022a). *SEIPS quick reference guide and work system explorer.* Available from: www.england.nhs.uk/wp-content/uploads/2022/08/B1465-SEIPS-quick-reference-and-work-system-explorer-v1-FINAL.pdf

NHS England. (2022b). *Patient safety learning response toolkit.* Available from: www.england.nhs.uk/publication/patient-safety-learning-response-toolkit

NHS Improvement. (2022). *Patient Safety Incident Response Framework Contributory and mitigating factors classification.* Available from: www.england.nhs.uk/wp-content/uploads/2020/08/PSII_Contributory_and_Mitigation_Factors_Classification.pdf

Shropshire Community Health NHS Trust. (n.d.). *Using stories to improve Patient, Carer and Staff experiences and outcomes.* Available from: www.england.nhs.uk/6cs/wp-content/uploads/sites/25/2015/09/scht-storytelling-toolkit.pdf

Sujan, M. A., Huang, H., & Braithwaite, J. (2017). Learning from incidents in health care: Critique from a Safety-II perspective. *Safety Science*, 99, 115–121.

The Health Foundation. (2011). *Improvement science.* Available from: www.health.org.uk/publications/improvement-science

US Department of Veterans Affairs. (2015). *Root Cause Analysis.* VA National Centre for Patient Safety. Available from: www.patientsafety.va.gov/media/rca.asp

World Health Organization. (2011). Patient Safety Curriculum Guide: Multi-Professional Edition. Geneva: WHO.

Wu, A. W., Lipshutz, A.K., & Pronovost, P. J. (2008). Effectiveness and efficiency of root cause analysis in medicine. *JAMA*, 299, 685–687.

# PART 3

# Investigating in diverse environments

# 9 Managing diversity and vulnerability

*Peggy Mulongo and John Wainwright*

## Introduction

It is important to recognise that the UK government's *Inclusive Britain* strategy underpins an action plan to create a fairer Britain which tackles unfair disparities and promotes unity (Gov.UK, 2021). It should go without saying that this attitude of fairness, equality, and justice needs to underpin everything that we do, for all. To do that, we need to be aware of the lived experience of those we are investigating, especially when they are vulnerable and unfamiliar with UK cultural norms. Hence, this chapter focuses on the challenges encountered by asylum-seeking men, women, and children in immigration removal centres (IRCs) in the UK immigration and the criminal justice system. In terms of justice, health, and inclusion, this population exemplifies a diverse and vulnerable population who are treated with suspicion and individually investigated regarding their right to remain. Their lives are 'on hold' pending the outcome of such an investigation. Whilst not every supported asylum seeker is vulnerable (Gov.UK, 2023), the UK government has a duty to protect the safety and wellbeing of those accommodated as refugees, and when incidents or harmful events occur, they also have a duty to investigate such events. This chapter aims to provide context and appreciation of the individual's experience and raise awareness of aligned legislation.

By examining the impact of immigration policies, institutional responses, and demographic realities, systemic failures perpetuating individual vulnerabilities will be discussed, focusing on two specific aspects: (i) asylum-seeking women detained in IRCs, restrictive and uncertain environments that pose significant challenges to the mental wellbeing of these women; (ii) challenges encountered by unaccompanied asylum-seeking children (UASC) in the UK immigration and the criminal justice system, particularly male asylum-seeking children. Despite efforts to safeguard the rights of male UASC, discrepancies in age assessments have engendered complexities in accessing suitable support and care (Age Assessment Task and Finish Group, 2015), affecting their health and education, and highlighting gender disparities in this particular group of immigrants.

Globally, over 100 million people have been forced to flee their homes, a number doubled compared to ten years ago, exceeding 100 million for the first time in 2022, with 35 per cent of this group being children and adolescents (UNHCR, 2023).

DOI: 10.4324/9781003286240-13

Refugees often experience traumatic events in their country of origin or during flight, including loss, separation, and sometimes even abuse (Kotovicz et al., 2018).

The UN Refugee Agency (UNHCR, 2019) identifies three durable solutions for the refugees: (i) return to their home country once security has been reestablished; (ii) integration into the country of first asylum, which is frequently a neighbouring country; (iii) resettlement in a different country, which is commonly high-income countries like the UK, USA, Canada, and Australia (Mulongo et al., 2021). Although resettlement seems to be the best option for refugees to find a safe environment in a foreign country, this poses new challenges as many refugees experience displacement, adjustment problems to the host country such as those related to language and communication, adaptation to a new culture and system, lack of support, discrimination, a loss of resources, and experience of trauma (González Campanella, 2023). For refugee status claimants (known as asylum seekers), the uncertainty of the claim process, lack of access to essential services, and sometimes detention upon arrival have been indicated as added stressors that could lead to retraumatisation (Marlowe, 2018).

### Differentiating the terms 'refugee' and 'asylum seeker'

The UN Convention describes a refugee as:

> a person who is outside his/her country of nationality or habitual residence; has a well-founded fear of persecution because of his/her race, religion, nationality, membership in a particular social group or political opinion [and is] unwilling to avail himself/herself of the protection of that country, or to return there, for fear of persecution.
>
> (United Nations 1951, p.152)

This global definition would include asylum seekers; however, an asylum claimant's case will be pending until a decision is made as to whether refugee status should be granted or not.

The UNHCR (2011) defines an asylum seeker as:

> An individual who has fled his/her country of origin to request sanctuary in another country, waiting for his/her claim to be processed.

Recognition for international protection as a refugee would depend on existing national asylum systems in countries where the person has sought asylum. Government members have the power to grant subsidiary protection to those who do not qualify under the UN Convention or reject individuals' asylum claims, with the risk of destitution or deportation (Refugee Council, 2014).

### Refugee resettlement programmes in the UK – the context

The United Kingdom (UK) has a remarkable history of being open to the world. Individuals can apply for asylum once they have entered the country regardless of how they entered. In the 21st century, UK immigration had been greater and of increasingly diverse origins than at any other point in its history, especially before Brexit and the COVID-19 pandemic in 2020. Also, the UK government has always prided itself on fulfilling its moral and legal responsibilities by supporting refugees fleeing peril around the world, and helping those facing persecution, oppression, and tyranny (Home Office, 2022). In 2021, the government said, 'as a force for good in the world', the UK would remain 'sensitive to the plight of refugees and asylum-seekers', having a 'proud track record' of protecting those who need it, in accordance with its international obligations (UK Parliament, 2022).

The above pledge, however, is contradictory to the recent government reform of the 'broken' UK asylum system in 2022 (UK Parliament, 2022). Whilst the UNHCR (2023) recognises the right for asylum seekers to be treated fairly and lawfully regardless of their race, gender, age, religion, sexual orientation, or any disability, newly implemented asylum policies actively discourage asylum seekers, including the 'four Ds of deterrence' – dispersal, detention, deportation, and destitution (Lewis et al., 2017) – and the recently adopted Illegal Migration Act (2023).

The latter has been a cause of concern for the United Nations (UN) Refugee Agency and UN Human Rights (UNHR) Office (Home Office, 2023b). The Illegal Migration Act 2023 stops people from seeking refugee protection or making other human rights claims in the UK, requiring their detention and prompt removal either to their home country or a safe third country, with no guarantee to access protection there, creating extensive new detention powers, with limited judicial oversight (UNHCR, 2023), accentuating the already existing stress and anxiety in this targeted population.

In 2022, the UK received 89,398 applications for asylum (including dependents). This is one-third of the number of applications received by Germany (243,835) and considerably fewer than France (156,455) and Spain (117,945) in the same period (Home Office, 2023b). This number slightly increased to 93,296 in September 2023 (Home Office, 2023b), which is still making a tiny proportion of new arrivals in the UK, whilst recognising that 6 per cent of the total asylum applications are from children who arrived in the UK alone without a parent or guardian, 16 per cent fewer than in 2022 (Home Office, 2023b). Around 43 per cent of people seeking asylum in the UK in 2020 were women and children (Home Office, 2023b).

Immigration policies have been criticised for failing to address human rights, and for their potential to emotionally, psychologically, and mentally harm vulnerable groups, including vulnerable groups of unaccompanied asylum-seeking children (UASC) and asylum-seeking women detained in IRCs (UNHCR, 2023; Pollard & Howard, 2021).

## Unaccompanied asylum-seeking children (UASC) in the UK – an uncertain status

Unaccompanied children, also known as unaccompanied minors, are children who have been separated from both parents and other relatives, and are not under the care of an adult who is legally or traditionally responsible for their wellbeing (Sanchez-Clemente et al., 2023).Common reasons prompting their departure often involve enduring harsh conditions such as hunger, restricted access to education and healthcare, low economic standing, and being exposed to violence, conflict, abuse, and exploitation (ISSOP, 2017).

In 2022, there were 5,242 applications from UASC cared for by local authorities; of these, 3,681 (70%) were aged 16 or 17. The latter age group is often disputed (Home Office, 2023b). Age-disputed cases are cases where an applicant claims to be a child but the Home Office assessment of appearance, or occasionally other evidence, leads to a dispute of the claim to be a child (Refugee Council, 2022). In other words, an immigration officer would decide on the case immigration status based on the young person's physical appearance and/or general behaviour, which 'very strongly indicates that they are 25 years or over' (Refugee Council, 2022). Unaccompanied children's claims are mainly granted refugee status where the decision is made whilst the child is under 18, but those who have reached the age of 18 when a decision is made are more likely to have their asylum claim refused (Refugee Council, 2022). Some of the unaccompanied children can be granted short-term leave to remain, which expires after 2.5 years, leaving them uncertain and anxious about their futures.

Forced migration presents distinct challenges for children and young refugees, exacerbating the negative effects of traumatic experiences. Various factors like gender, age, and nationality, significantly impact their mental health, especially amongst unaccompanied asylum-seeking children (Lopez-Murray, 2019; Müller et al., 2019). In the UK, children under 14 years old arrive seeking safety and protection. Whilst some receive full asylum status, others might get short-term leave lasting 2.5 years, causing uncertainty and anxiety if full status isn't granted upon expiration. Despite the UK government's pledge in 2010 to end child detention practices, these persist, with 57 children held in immigration detention by September 2023, raising concerns about potential increases under the Illegal Migration Act 2023 (Home Office, 2023a). Although the Secretary of State isn't obliged to arrange a child's removal from the UK until they reach 18 years old, there exists the authority to do so (Home Office, 2023b).

By incorporating gender perspectives, age disputes, and criminal justice into the discussion of this chapter, the authors highlight the nuanced challenges, prevalent health issues, and barriers to accessing mental health support for male UASC within the UK healthcare system. The critical discussion underscores the importance of recognising male gender-specific vulnerabilities and integrating gender-sensitive approaches into care provisions for male UASC.

## Unaccompanied asylum-seeking children (UASC) in the UK – gender perspectives

The literature demonstrates a high level of vulnerability for female UASC to develop poor mental health due to traumatic incidents of physical and sexual violence during the different phases of the migration process, compared to their male counterpart (Mohwinkel et al., 2018). It is suggested that female refugee children, when compared to those accompanied by at least one parent, may face a higher risk of developing post-traumatic stress disorder (PTSD) and depression within the context of forced migration and settlement (Hazer & Gredebäck, 2023).

Female and male UASC may have different reasons to flee their home countries. Risks of violence and abuse experienced may be gender-specific, such as recruitment as child soldiers for boys or forced marriage for girls, making it difficult to compare the degree of vulnerability, based on gender.

Perceptions regarding male UASC have evolved over time, and one approach to comprehending how these perspectives arise is by considering them as stemming from two conflicting storylines. One storyline portrays them as vulnerable children requiring safeguarding, whilst the other depicts them as dangerous and delinquent youths (Lems et al., 2020), the latter having become the dominant narrative over time. Having initially been described in the media as vulnerable, traumatised, and in need of help, they increasingly came to be depicted as criminal young males who had lied about their age in order to exploit the welfare systems of receiving countries, and who constituted a threat to public order (Lems et al., 2020). Furthermore, findings from the study conducted by Pettersson and Vogel (2023) show that assessments of problems experienced by male UASC follow common gender patterns for some, whilst for others they are more similar to assessments focused on girls. Furthermore, Pettersson and Vogel (2023) found that less focus was placed on the educational careers of UASC under compulsory care, either because of restricted schooling requirements (due to their age and/or their refugee status) or because they entered the country after the school term had started, being subject to frequent dispersal in different areas and making continuous school attendance more difficult.

Schools can represent a safe place for refugee children. However, being a minor and looking mature is a challenging issue for male UASC in school, and few studies present age-adjusted results on gender differences (Keles et al., 2016) in this particular group of youths, where higher age is associated with higher PTSD scores (Smid et al., 2011).

Wood et al. (2020) highlight that male UASC may encounter heightened vulnerability to violence, exploitation, struggles with masculine identities during displacement, and gender-related trauma including conflict-induced violence. Conversely, the experiences of female UASC often involve distinct challenges related to gender-based violence, exploitation, and reproductive health concerns (Wood et al., 2020).

## Mental health issues

There is evidence that the asylum process impacts on mental health for UASC, the majority of whom are boys or young men (Home Office, 2019).

Many refugee youths suffer from PTSD and related mental health problems, such as anxiety, depression, paranoia, and personality disorders (Frounfelker et al, 2020; Miller et al., 2018). Post-resettlement, depression and anxiety were consistently high amongst USAC and associated with discrimination, limited language attainment, and daily hassles (Bamford et al., 2021).

Comorbid PTSD, depression, and anxiety are the most prevalent disorders amongst UASC in Europe (Bamford et al., 2021). The increased vulnerability to developing mental health problems is assumed to be due to several risk factors, including separation from parents, a high exposure to potentially traumatic events, and the loss of their familiar environment and support system, whilst being faced with the continuous stressors associated with migration (Demazure et al., 2018).

Safety (serious) incidents that occur outside of the NHS do not come under the Patient Safety Incident Response Framework (PSIRF) as such, but they are covered by a safeguarding framework that enables investigation in case of adverse incidents. The factors contributing to safety incidents in mental health care for UASMC are multifaceted and contribute to increasing the risk of poorer outcomes following exposure to adverse childhood experiences (ACEs). Overcrowding, insufficient resources, and prolonged waiting times within mental healthcare facilities (Wood et al., 2020) exacerbate vulnerabilities, contributing to incidents of self-harm, suicidal behaviours, physical assaults or neglect. Additionally, the intersection of legal complexities, particularly related to age disputes, further compounds distress, hindering timely mental health interventions.

### Conducting investigations within the context of cultural diversity and vulnerability

Whilst acknowledging the importance of cultural awareness and respect of the other person, it is most often language differences that are likely to create a challenge when conducting an investigative interview (Benuto & Garrick, 2016); hence, working well with an interpreter is pivotal to a successful interview. Accessing an interpreter can be a challenge, but Benuto and Garrick (2016) warn not to be tempted to use family or friends in this role. Walsh et al. (2020) highlighted a number of areas where we can enhance the success of interpreter-assisted interviews, including the joint planning of the interview, with the interpreter building and maintaining a rapport with the interviewee. Chapter 6 speaks at length about conducting an investigative interview and the utilisation of the PEACE model, and these foundational principles can still be adopted while applying culturally sensitive interviewing (Muniroh et al, 2018).

### Conclusion

In focusing on distinct, albeit minority groups, we have attempted to raise awareness of the experience of cultural diversity and vulnerability in the context of investigation. UK legislation has been considered as well as research that can guide us in the rights and struggles of this population, as well as informative practice that can aid us in our approach.

### References

Age Assessment Task and Finish Group (2015) *Guidance to assist social workers and their managers in undertaking age assessments in England.* The Association of Directors of Children's Services. Available from: https://adcs.org.uk/assets/documentation/Age_Assessment_Guidance_2015_Final.pdf

Bamford, J., Fletcher, M., & Leavey, G. (2021). Mental health outcomes of unaccompanied refugee minors: A rapid review of recent research. *Current Psychiatry Reports*, 23(8), 46.

Benuto, L. T., & Garrick, J. (2016). Cultural considerations in forensic interviewing of children. In W. T. Donohue & M. Fanetti (eds), *Forensic Interviews Regarding Child Sexual Abuse: A Guide to Evidence-Based Practice* (pp.351–364). Springer.

Demazure, G., Gaultier, S., & Pinsault, N. (2018). Dealing with difference: A scoping review of psychotherapeutic interventions with unaccompanied refugee minors. *European Child & Adolescent Psychiatry*, 27, 447–466.

Frounfelker, R. L., Miconi, D., Farrar, J., Brooks, M. A., Rousseau, C., & Betancourt, T. S. (2020). mental health of refugee children and youth: epidemiology, interventions, and future directions. *Annual Review of Public Health*, 41, 159–176. https://doi.org/10.1146/annurev-publhealth-040119-094230

González Campanella, A. (2023). Availability and acceptability of interpreting services for refugees as a question of trauma-informed care. *Interpreting and Society*, 3(1), 75–94.

Gov.UK. (2021). Inclusive Britain: government response to the Commission on Race and Ethnic Disparities. Available from: www.gov.uk/government/publications/inclusive-britain-action-plan-government-response-to-the-commission-on-race-and-ethnic-disparities

Gov.UK. (2022). New Plan for Immigration: policy statement. Available from: www.gov.uk/government/consultations/new-plan-for-immigration/new-plan-for-immigration-policy-statement-accessible

Hazer, L., & Gredebäck, G. (2023). The effects of war, displacement, and trauma on child development. Humanities and Social Sciences Communications, 10, 909.

Home Office. (2022). *Asylum interviews.* Available from: https://assets.publishing.service.gov.uk/government/uploads/system/uploads/attachment_data/file/1176830/Asylum_interview.pdf

Home Office. (2023a). Illegal Migration Act 2023. Available from: www.gov.uk/government/collections/illegal-migration-bill

Home Office (Gov.UK) (2023b). National statistics: Immigration system statistics, year ending September 2023. Statistics relating to the operation of the immigration system, including visas, extensions, citizenship, asylum, resettlement, detention and returns. Available from: www.gov.uk/government/statistics/immigration-system-statistics-year-ending-september-2023

International Society for Social Pediatrics and Child Health (ISSOP). (2017). ISSOP position statement on migrant child health. *Child Care Health and Developement*, 44(1), 161–170.

Keles, S., Friborg, O., Idsøe, T., et al. (2016). Depression among unaccompanied minor refugees: The relative contribution of general and acculturation-specific daily hassles. *Ethnicity & Health.* 21(3), 300–317.

Kotovicz, F., Getzin, A., & Vo, T. (2018). Challenges of refugee health care: Perspectives of medical interpreters, case managers, and pharmacists. Journal of Patient-Centered Research and Reviews, 5(1), 28.

Lems, A., Oester, K., & Strasser, S. (2020). Children of the crisis: Ethnographic perspectives on unaccompanied refugee youth in and en route to Europe. *Journal of Ethnic and Migration Studies*, 46(2), 315–335.

Lewis, H., Waite, L., & Hodkinson, S. (2017). 'Hostile' UK Immigration Policy and Asylum Seekers' Susceptibility to Forced Labour. In F.Vecchio & A. Gerard (eds). *Entrapping Asylum Seekers: Transnational Crime, Crime Control and Security.* London: Palgrave Macmillan.

Lopez-Murray, E. (2019). Health of asylum-seeking immigrants: Providing medical care from a volunteer's perspective. *JAAPA*, 32(8), 13–14.

Marlowe, J. (2018). *Belonging and Transnational Refugee Settlement: Unsettling the Everyday and the Extraordinary.* London: Taylor & Francis.

Miller, A., Hess, J. M., Bybee, D., & Goodkind, J. R. (2018). Understanding the mental health consequences of family separation for refugees: Implications for policy and practice. *American Journal of Orthopsychiatry*, 88(1), 26–37. https://doi.org/10.1037/ort0000272

Milne, R., Bull, R. (1999). Investigative *Interviewing: Psychology* and *Practice*. Chichester: Wiley.

Mohwinkel, L. M., Nowak, A. C., Kasper, A., & Razum, O. (2018). Gender differences in the mental health of unaccompanied refugee minors in Europe: A systematic review. *BMJ Open*, 8(7).

Müller, L. R. F., Büter, K. P., Rosner, R., & Unterhitzenberger, J. (2019). Mental health and associated stress factors in accompanied and unaccompanied refugee minors resettled in Germany: A cross-sectional study. *Child and Adolescent Psychiatry and Mental Health*, 13, Article 8. https://doi.org/10.1186/s13034-019-0268-1

Mulongo, P., McAndrew, S., & Ayodeji, E. (2021). Resettling into a new life: Exploring aspects of acculturation that could enhance the mental health of young refugees resettled under the humanitarian programme. *International Journal of Mental Health Nursing*, 30, 235–248. https://doi.org/10.1111/inm.12777

Muniroh, R. D. D., Findling, J., & Heydon, G. (2018). What's in a question: A case for a culturally appropriate interviewing protocol in the Australian Refugee Review Tribunal. In I. M. Nick (ed.) *Forensic Linguistics, Asylum Seekers, Refugees and Immigrants* (pp.133–154). Vernon Press.

Pettersson, T., & Vogel, M. A. (2023). Compulsory care placements among unaccompanied male refugee minors. *Nordic Journal of Criminology*, 24(1), 1–22.

Pollard, T., & Howard, N. (2021). Mental healthcare for asylum-seekers and refugees residing in the United Kingdom: A scoping review of policies, barriers, and enablers. *International Journal of Mental Health Systems*, 15, 60.

Refugee Council (2014). Briefing for debate on 29 January 2014: The UK's participation in the United Nations High Commissioner for Refugees (UNHCR) Syrian Refugees Programme. Amnesty International and Refugee Council.

Refugee Council (2022). *Children in the Asylum System.* Asylum statistics published quarterly by the Home Office.

Sanchez-Clemente, N., Eisen, S., Harkensee, C., Longley, N., O'Grady, R., & Ward, A. (2023). Beyond arrival: Safeguarding unaccompanied asylum-seeking children in the UK. *Archives of Disease in Childhood*, 108(3), 160–165.

Smid, G. E., Lensvelt-Mulders, G. J., Knipscheer, J. W., et al. (2011). Late-onset PTSD in unaccompanied refugee minors: Exploring the predictive utility of depression and anxiety symptoms. *Journal of Clinical Child and Adolesc Psychology*, 40(5), 742–755.

UK Parliament. (2022). Refugees and asylum-seekers: UK policy. House of Lords Library. Available from: https://lordslibrary.parliament.uk/refugees-and-asylum-seekers-uk-policy/#heading-8

United Nations. (1951). *Convention Relating to the Status of Refugees*. Geneva: United Nations General Assesmbly.

UNHCR. (2011). Handbook and Guidelines on Procedures and Criteria for Determining Refugee Status under the 1951 Convention and the 1967 Protocol Relating to the Status of Refugees. Available from: www.unhcr.org/uk/media/handbook-procedures-and-criteria-determining-refugee-status-under-1951-convention-and-1967

UNHCR. (2023). UK Asylum and Policy and the Illegal Migration Act. Available from: www.unhcr.org/uk/what-we-do/uk-asylum-and-policy-and-illegal-migration-act/uk-asylum-and-policy-and-illegal

UN Refugee Agency. (2019). Global trends. Forced displacement in 2019. Available from: www.unhcr.org/media/unhcr-global-trends-2019

Walsh, D., Oxburgh, G. E., & Amurun, T. (2020). Interpreter-assisted interviews: Examining investigators' and interpreters' views on their practice. *Journal of Police and Criminal Psychology*, 35, 318–327.

Wood, S., Ford, K., Hardcastle, K., Hopkins, J., Hughes, K., & Bellis, M. A; (2020). *Adverse Childhood Experiences in child refugee and asylum-seeking populations.* Cardiff: Public Health Wales NHS Trust.

# 10 Serious incident investigations involving children and young people

*Louise Hamer and Tim McDougall*

## Introduction

This chapter will explore how serious incident investigations involving children and young people differ from those involving adults. Case examples will be included to illustrate how the processes operate and interact between the NHS and local authority children's services. The importance of children's rights and capturing the child's voice and that of their parents in serious incident investigations will be discussed, recognising their inherent vulnerability from a sociology of childhood perspective.

A central focus throughout the chapter will be on safeguarding. As part of Working Together to Safeguard Children (Department for Education, 2015) the processes in incidents which involve death or serious harm to a child, where abuse or neglect is known or suspected, and deaths of children in care and children in regulated settings will be discussed.

There will be an overview of how safeguarding boards operate and discharge their statutory functions in relation to oversight and learning from serious incidents and their role in holding partner organisations to account. How professionals and agencies work with parents and carers, schools, and wider children's services partners will be discussed.

As with serious incident investigations in general, the aim of those involving children and young people is to identify the factors that may have contributed in order to help prevent future harm. This is particularly important from a perspective of safeguarding and child protection where preventative strategies and interventions may limit or reduce harm to children looked after by their parents, carers, or the state.

When undertaking any review of a serious safeguarding incident involving children and young people, it is important to first understand the context within which the incident has occurred. For children and young people, *context* relates to a range of political, social, and individual factors that coexist in a child's life, creating an environment where harm can occur. By considering context in this way, it is possible to understand how serious incident investigations involving children and young people differ fundamentally from those involving adults. Political, social,

DOI: 10.4324/9781003286240-14

and individual child factors are all important to take into consideration and are discussed throughout this chapter.

### How often do serious incidents involving children occur?

Notifiable serious incidents are those that involve death or serious harm to a child where abuse or neglect is known or suspected, and any death of a looked-after child (HM Government, 2023). These incidents are reported by local authorities to child safeguarding practice review (CSPR) panels and are monitored by the Department for Education in England. During the financial year of 2021–2022 a total of 442 serious incident notifications were made by local authorities in relation to children, of which 191 involved the death of a child (HM Government, 2023).

Whilst approximately 42 per cent of deaths involve children aged less than one and relate to unsafe sleeping practices (National Child Mortality Database, 2022), most serious incident investigations in mental health services which directly involve children and young people are a result of death following an attempt to end life. Suicide is the third leading cause of death for both girls and boys aged 15–19 (World Health Organization, 2019). However, whether investigations conclude that a child or young person's death was a result of suicide is a matter for coroners. For mental health and other services, the objective is to review the circumstances which led to the death with a view to learning lessons and preventing future deaths. Depending on the agencies involved and the circumstances in which the child or young people died, there may be parallel serious incident reviews and child safeguarding practice reviews.

The National Confidential Inquiry in Suicide and Safety in Mental Health (NCISH) produces periodic thematic reports into reviews of deaths by children and young and people. The most recent of these (NCISH, 2023) examined 391 deaths of children and young people in England and Wales. The review identified parental mental illness or substance misuse; childhood abuse; bullying; physical health; mental ill-health; and alcohol or drug misuse as themes. Key learning is published in relation to identifying children and young people at risk; suicide related internet use; self-harm; and the need for age-appropriate interventions (NCISH, 2023).

### Political factors

A number of high-profile incidents involving serious harm and death of children have framed the political climate in which investigations take place. The depth, quality, and influence of these investigations has evolved considerably over time. The regulatory framework for children's services also provides a context in which investigations take place. In England, children's social care services are inspected by Ofsted and children's health services are inspected by the Care Quality Commission. Both regulators are government funded and so are influenced by the politics of the day.

### Case example: Jasmine Beckford – 1984

Jasmine Beckford was four years old when she was murdered by her step-father in July 1984. Jasmine had spent periods of time in local authority foster care before being returned to her mother's care. During the inquiry that followed, Jasmine's social worker said 'the family obviously loved the children' but admitted only seeing Jasmine once in ten months, believing the family's explanations as to why she was unavailable. The reality was that Jasmine had experienced high levels of violence during that time and had up to 40 different injuries recorded at the time of her death.

Widespread reform of the child protection system in England and Wales came in the form of the Children Act (1989) after Jasmine's death. One of the central findings of the Beckford Inquiry into the case of Jasmine Beckford (London Borough of Brent, 1985) was that professionals had considered the parents of children in care as their primary clients rather than the child in their own right. As a result, the principle that the welfare of the child is paramount became embedded in law within the Children Act (1989). Although the principle has no direct application outside a court setting, the best interests of a child must always be a guiding consideration for children's professionals and staff. Any intervention from the state should be child focused, and the child's right to be protected from harm should supersede all other considerations.

### Case example: Victoria Climbié

Victoria Climbié was an eight-year-old girl who died in 2000 in Haringey, North London. Victoria had moved to the UK from the Ivory Coast to live with her great-aunt around 18 months earlier, her parents believing they were sending her to 'live a better life'. The reality was Victoria suffered a cata-logue of abuse over an 11-month period whilst in the care of her great-aunt and had 128 different injuries reported at the time of her death. Sadly, Victoria had come to the attention of services in the preceding 12 months includ-ing the police, children's social care and health, but the system had failed to keep her safe.

The Victoria Climbié Inquiry was undertaken by Lord Laming in 2003. It con-cluded that her abuse did not take place out of sight or behind closed doors, but that Victoria had been, 'abandoned, unheard and unnoticed by the very system designed to protect her' (Laming, 2003). Laming declared that whilst the child protection system had failed Victoria catastrophically, the fundamental fault was in the application of the Children Act (1989). Laming criticised the system as grossly underfunded and scarcely resourced, and he proposed that children were not afforded the same level of investigation by the police as adults who had suffered similar harm.

Following Lord Laming's review into the death of Victoria Climbié came the revision of the Children Act (1989) which was amended in 2004. This was mirrored by a government policy called Every Child Matters (HM Treasury, 2003) which was significant not only in reforming systems and processes within child protection, but also in challenging the way that children were considered within society at that time. In the policy introduction, Paul Boateng, the then Chief Secretary to the Treasury, noted that 'underpinning reform is not just about resources but an attitude that reflects the value that our society places on children and childhood' (HM Treasury, 2003).

Following the 2004 amendment of the Children Act (1989), the state maintained responsibility for protecting children at risk of or experiencing significant harm but Every Child Matters introduced a new discourse and strapline that safeguarding children was 'everybody's business'. A children's commissioner for England was established to lead on the children's rights agenda and local safeguarding children boards (LSCBs) were established. These LSCBs were given statutory responsibility for undertaking multi-agency serious case reviews (SCRs) when there was reason to believe a child had died or been seriously injured as a result of abuse or neglect.

A Common Assessment Framework was developed and introduced to standardise assessment of children and family need across all agencies including health, education, police, and children's social care. As Haringey in North London was reported to be in the top 10 per cent of most deprived areas of the country at the time of Victoria Climbié's death, links began to be made between levels of community deprivation and children suffering significant harm. There was recognition that poverty and disadvantage impacted negatively on a child's health and wellbeing, and that not all children and communities were created equal.

Every Child Matters (HM Treasury, 2003) made a clear and fundamental distinction between *child protection* and *safeguarding children*. Significant harm remained the threshold for statutory child protection intervention under section 47 of the Children Act (1989) and the point at which local authorities had a duty to investigate to enable them to decide whether action was required to safeguard or promote a child's welfare. However, the wider safeguarding agenda through Every Child Matters reinforced the moral and professional responsibility to *all* children who were entitled to a basic human right to live safely, free from abuse and neglect, as set out in article 19 of the United Nations Convention on Rights of the Child (UNICEF 1989). Every Child Matters extended the responsibility for keeping children safe beyond the family home and individual parents to the wider community. Safeguarding reviews were thus required to consider the wider context in which children live.

**Case example: Peter Connelly – 2013**

Peter Connelly (Baby P) was just 17 months old when he died whilst in the care of his mother and her partner and lodger in Haringey, North London, in 2007. Peter had suffered 50 different injuries, including a broken back at the time of his death. Investigations undertaken by the Metropolitan Police in relation to the non-accidental injury of Peter when he was nine and 12 months old had not resulted in any criminal prosecution and Peter remained in his mother's care. Like Victoria Climbié, Peter had not been invisible to services and had been seen by social workers, police, and health professionals around 60 times in the final eight months of his life (Haringey LSCB, 2008).

At the time of Peter Connelly's death, the aim of a serious case review (SCR) (as of 2018 referred to as a child safeguarding practice review) was to identify and establish learning for agencies and professionals with a view to improving the way they work independently and together to safeguard children. The recommendations made by Lord Laming just a few years earlier following Victoria Climbié's death and the policy aspirations of Every Child Matters (HM Treasury, 2003) had failed to keep Peter safe. The SCR into his death identified staff shortages, poor communication, and poor leadership within children's social care as contributory factors.

In 2011, Eileen Munro was asked by the then Secretary of State for Education, Michael Gove, to conduct an independent review of child protection in England. This was due to growing concerns that the system had become overly bureaucratised and focused on compliance, and needed to be more child centred. Munro's findings did not lead to any changes to the Children Act (1989) but Working Together to Safeguard Children (Department for Education, 2013) was revised. Amongst the revisions was the formal introduction of the 'early help' agenda. This was in recognition that early intervention and family support were essential in supporting the most vulnerable children. There was a restated need for shared responsibility between local authorities, police, education, and health, alongside a reinforced need to share information. Agencies were required to work together and protect children from experiencing escalating levels of harm, built on the foundations of the Common Assessment Framework introduced by Every Child Matters in 2003 (HM Treasury, 2003).

Whilst section 47 of the Children Act (1989) introduced the concept of significant harm as the threshold for statutory child protection intervention in England and Wales, there was no nationally agreed criteria as to what significant harm entailed. Local safeguarding children boards were instructed to define what significant harm meant to their local population of children, identify levels of harm towards children along a 'continuum of need' (see Figure 10.1 below) and publish local guidance in the form of a multi-agency threshold document. Figure 10.2 below is an example of how the local authority in which the authors work has described the continuum of need as guidance for staff and partner organisations (Children's Safeguarding and Assurance Partnership, 2021).

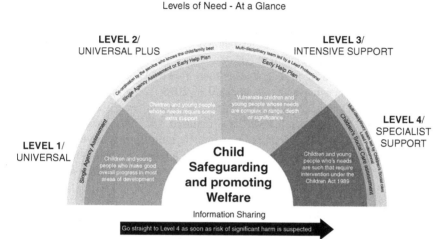

*Figure 10.1* Continuum of Need (Lancashire model)

The concept of significant harm, as opposed to a national definition, enabled a degree of subjectivity in how the term was understood to flourish. What constitutes significant harm can differ greatly between local authority areas. This leads to inconsistency in how statutory child protection thresholds are applied for children and young people living in different parts of the country.

## The Wood Review – 2016

Local safeguarding children boards have been responsible for the commissioning of Serious Case Reviews since 2013. Since that time, the Department for Education has been responsible for conducting triennial reviews of SCRs to undertake thematic analysis and share learning nationally across the safeguarding system. This is again with the aim of avoiding similar serious incidents occurring. The most recent triennial review considered learning from SCRs which took place between 2014 and 2017 (Department for Education, 2020) and found that 1.3 children die in England and Wales every week as a result of abuse or neglect. The review concluded that the number of SCRs completed following the death of a child has been consistent over time, but the number in relation to serious harm has increased when compared to the previous three years (Department for Education, 2020).

In 2016, Alan Wood, a former director of children's services in London, was asked to undertake a strategic review of the role and function of LSCBs. The concern was that despite repeated reform (Laming, 2003; HM Treasury, 2003; Munro,

2011; Department for Education, 2013), very little appeared to have changed for children and young people at risk of abuse and neglect. With each SCR predicted to cost between £5,000 and £30,000 (Kingston et al., 2018), the system was proving expensive and difficult to sustain. One of the recommendations made by the Wood Review (Department for Education (England), 2016) was that time-consuming and costly SCRs should be replaced by child safeguarding practice reviews (CSPRs) and that they would be triggered by a so-called 'rapid review', completed within 15 working days of a child being harmed.

The introduction of rapid reviews was supported by Working Together to Safeguard Children when it was again updated in 2018 (Department for Education, 2018). The aim of safeguarding partnerships was to identify early learning and consider whether a more in-depth CSPR was required. Crucially, local safeguarding partnerships were no longer required to complete multi-agency reviews for every child that had died or been seriously harmed (as a result of abuse and neglect) if they could evidence similar learning had been identified by an earlier review.

### Case example: Arthur and Star – 2022

Arthur Laninjo-Jones, aged six, and Star Hobson, aged 16 months were two children tragically murdered by their caregivers in 2020. The children lived in different parts of the country (Solihull and Bradford), but both cases were heavily reported in the media. Arthur was murdered by his father's girlfriend and had been poisoned, starved, and beaten in the weeks before his death, and Star was murdered by her mother's girlfriend and had suffered psychological and physical abuse throughout her short life. Both children had suffered significant abuse and neglect, being surrounded by professionals and family members, yet the safeguarding system had been unable to keep them safe at the same time, causing national outrage in December 2021.

In January 2022, the National Child Safeguarding Practice Review Panel was commissioned to undertake a review into the circumstances leading up to the deaths of Arthur and Star. Sadly, their experiences were not unusual. Approximately one child is killed every week, with those under the age of one being the most at risk (Child Safeguarding Practice Review Panel, 2022). The panel made a number of recommendations for the child protection system. One of the most significant was a need to refocus on child protection within the safeguarding context. There is recognition that whilst safeguarding is everybody's business as set out in previous policy and strategy, child protection is a more focused area of health and social care practice, and requires an enhanced level of skill and expertise (Child Safeguarding Practice Review Panel, 2022).

### Social factors

Concepts of childhood, child protection, and safeguarding as well as what it means to be a child have evolved over time and across cultures. Politically and socially, this has shaped the safeguarding system at a national and local level, and influenced the way in which we respond to children. Derbyshire Safeguarding Children Board (2018) published an independent inquiry into the experiences of children and young people at Aston Hall in Derbyshire between the 1950s and 1970s. The report described children being drugged, sexually assaulted, and restrained using straitjackets. This so-called treatment centre closed with only passing public attention in 2004, which could be said to reflect attitudes to state-funded care of children at the time. The Cleveland Inquiry (Butler-Sloss, 1987) and the abuse of children in care in Wales (Department of Health, 2000) each highlighted abuse by staff who were charged with their care.

## The Children Act (1989)

The Children Act (1989) is the single most important piece of legislation for safeguarding children, providing the framework for statutory child protection in England and Wales. Along with human rights legislation, the Children Act (1989) provides the key legal framework governing the care and welfare of all children and young people under 18. The Children Act (1989) was passed in order to bring private and public law provisions in a single legislative framework affecting children and families. It attempts to balance the rights of children, the responsibilities of parents to their child and the duty of statutory agencies to intervene when concerns about the child's welfare requires them to do so.

Since 1989 there has been an evolving body of research and literature which points to childhood as a social construct, one that is influenced by historical and cultural factors rather than a homogenous stage of life defined by age alone (Prout & James, 1997; King 2007; Gallacher & Gallagher, 2008). When the Children Act was introduced in 1989, the role of the nuclear family was valued and seen as crucial in instilling values of decency, manners, respect for law, and developing self-reliance amongst British citizens (Page, 2015). Adults had previously been considered as superior to children (Speier, 1976, cited in Leonard, 2016), and there was a common law presumption that parents were entitled to moral rights in respect of their children as well as responsibility for them (Featherstone et al., 2018). Children were considered the property of parents, and a statutory duty to protect children from harm was founded on the belief that parents should be able to care for their own children as they saw fit.

Section 47 of the Children Act (1989) introduced the concept of significant harm as the threshold for statutory child protection. According to S47, local authorities are required to 'make enquiries where there is reasonable cause to suspect that a child who lives, or is found, in their area is suffering, or likely to suffer, significant harm'. The use of language in the Children Act (1989) definition is highly subjective and has introduced a discourse in child protection that *some* harm towards children is acceptable within the confines of family life. According to the legal framework, there has to be a *reasonable* cause for concern and the child has to be *likely* to suffer *significant* harm. What is classed as reasonable, likely or significant is locally determined by the children's safeguarding partnerships (Department for Education, 2018). This means there is variation across the country in relation to how thresholds for statutory child protection are applied and which children are protected by statutory agencies including the police, children's social care, and multi-agency safeguarding hubs (MASH).

Whilst the Children Act (1989) has since been amended by the Children (Leaving Care) Act (2000), the Adoption and Children Act (2002) and the Children Act (2004), the original Act remains in use today and its guiding principles should underpin all serious incident investigations involving children and young people.

## The United Nations Convention on the Rights of the Child (1989)

The United Nations Convention on the Rights of the Child (UNCRC) is of great significance as it recognised the inherent vulnerability of children in the form of a human rights treaty for the first time. It identified 54 civil, political, economic, social, and cultural rights for all children and young people across the world and was ratified by the UK in 1991. The articles of the UNCRC do not stand alone and should never be considered in isolation. Rather, the treaty should be viewed as a collection of articles which interact to create a framework that embeds children's rights into everyday life. The UNCRC and the Children Act (1989) entitle children to participatory decision-making rights. As children and young people become older and move towards independence, their involvement in matters that affect them should increase. Whatever the age of the child, it is always important to keep them as fully informed and involved as possible in the process of serious incident investigations. They should receive clear and detailed information in a format that is suitable to their age and developmental understanding.

A child's basic human right to be protected from harm is enshrined in article 19. Governments must do all they can to ensure that children are protected from all forms of violence, abuse, neglect, and bad treatment by their parents or anyone else who looks after them (UNICEF, 1989). Importantly from a safeguarding perspective, article 19 should be considered alongside article 12, which is the right to participate. Under article 12, children have a basic human right to express a view in all matters that affect them and for that view to be listened to and acted on as appropriate in line with their age and maturity. What article 12 introduced to the UK was recognition that a child was a full person with integrity, personality, and agency (Freeman, 1996). With article 12 came a belief that children were not passive but active participants in their own world with an ability to influence and shape their experiences.

Whilst the Children Act was revised in 2004, the key aspects of the legal framework have remained unchanged for over 30 years. There has been no update made following the introduction of the Care Act (2014) to align language with the adult safeguarding agenda, nor has there been any reflection of the children's rights agenda (UNCRC 1989) since it was ratified in 1991.

## The Care Act (2014)

The Care Act (2014) outlines the threshold for statutory intervention from an adult safeguarding perspective. In contrast to the Children Act (1989), it requires local authorities to make enquiries 'where there is reasonable cause to suspect that an adult (with care and support needs) is at risk of abuse or neglect'. Unlike with children, there is no requirement for vulnerable adults to be at risk of *significant* harm before the state has a duty to intervene; there simply needs to be a reasonable cause to suspect *risk of* abuse and neglect.

## Working Together to Safeguard Children (Department for Education, 2018)

The Children and Social Work Act (2017) introduced a new legal framework in respect of local safeguarding arrangements for children. Responsibility for how the safeguarding system was to learn lessons from serious incidents now rested at national level with the Child Safeguarding Practice Review Panel, and at local level with the safeguarding partnership. According to Working Together to Safeguard Children (Department of Education, 2018), three statutory partners make up a local safeguarding partnership, and these are health, police, and the local authority. It is Working Together to Safeguard Children (2018) that provides guidance to local safeguarding partnerships about when to undertake a child safeguarding practice review (CSPR). When the language of Working Together to Safeguard Children is considered alongside guidance provided by the Care Act (2014) in relation to safeguarding adult reviews, the difference between child and adult serious incident investigations becomes clear.

According to the Care Act (2014), the safeguarding adult board considers a serious safeguarding incident to be one where an adult with care and support needs:

a) has died and there are concerns that the death resulted from abuse or neglect.
b) has not died but there are concerns the adult has experienced abuse and neglect and there is reasonable cause or concern about how partner agencies have worked together to safeguard the adult.

In contrast, according to Working Together to Safeguard Children (2018) criteria, a serious safeguarding incident is where:

a) abuse or neglect of a child is known or suspected and;
b) the child has died or been seriously harmed. Seriously harmed being where a child has suffered serious and/or long-term impairment of their mental health or intellectual, emotional, social or behavioural development.

The line between what is and is not serious can be blurred and is always a matter of judgement. It depends on many factors, including age of the child, frequency of the incident, injuries sustained, any additional needs the child has. In some instances, the cumulative effect of frequent incidents may make a notification appropriate even if in isolation each event would not warrant this.

Children are required to experience harm more significantly than their adult counterparts to trigger a statutory protection response and must also suffer serious or long-term impairment before the criteria are met for safeguarding partnerships to undertake a multi-agency safeguarding review. Considering the language of the legal frameworks (Children Act 1989; Care Act 2014) alongside national guidance (Department for Education, 2018), the social context described by Speier (cited in Leonard, 2016), where adults are superior to children, appears to exist in the present day.

### Individual factors

The purpose of a child safeguarding practice review (CSPR) is not an enquiry about how a child has died or was seriously harmed or into who was culpable. Such questions will be addressed by coroners and criminal courts. Nor is a CSPR an investigation into individual staff and their actions or omissions. These matters are usually dealt with under the disciplinary or capability procedures of individual agencies. Rather, the aim of a CSPR is to identify learning at local and national level, and identify improvements which need to be made to the safeguarding system in order to promote the welfare of children.

Understanding where there are systemic issues and identifying how policy and practice need to change is crucial to the system being dynamic and self-improving. Reviews should seek to prevent or reduce the risk of recurrence of similar incidents, but the intention is not to hold individuals, organisations of agencies to account. It is not unusual for there to be parallel investigations taking place – for example, disciplinary procedures, professional regulation or criminal proceedings. It is important for the review to be aware of these at the outset so the terms of reference for any multi-agency review can be clear, child focused, and centred on learning.

There is no single prescribed methodology for conducting a multi-agency safeguarding review. Traditional serious case reviews have been process driven, and there has been a range of different models utilised by different safeguarding boards across the UK (Kingston et al., 2018). According to Working Together to Safeguard Children (Department for Education, 2018), safeguarding children partnerships should be able to choose the review methodology that is suitable for their local arrangements. Some examples include:

- **Root cause analysis (RCA):** The use of systematic analysis to explore beyond individual involvement in a case and understand the underlying causes to establish how or why an incident took place.
- **Significant incident learning process (SILP):** This is a whole-systems approach which directly hears the voice of frontline practitioners involved in critical events; examines how their interaction with different workplace systems affects understanding, decision making, and action; and explores how these different systems interact across agency boundaries. The investigative process was developed by Review Consulting after recommendations made by the Munro report (2011). It includes a review of agency reports aligned to 'critical incidents' followed by a practitioner 'learning event' and 'recall session'.

- **Appreciative inquiry (AI):** This is a strengths-based, positive approach to organisational learning and change. The method seeks to create a safe, supportive environment to highlight the positive aspects of a case alongside the challenges. The focus is around moving forward, and the investigative process is underpinned by solution focused techniques.
- **The Welsh model:** This describes the child practice review framework developed in Wales in 2015. The review process aims to be more focused and begins with the formation of a multi-agency timeline. The timeline only includes significant events in the 12 months leading up to a serious incident taking place. The focus of the review is multi-agency learning for current practice and aims to be completed within a six-month period. Similar to other review methodology, there is a practitioner learning event held by an independent reviewer, and practitioners are invited to speak in a safe space about the reality of their safeguarding work.

It remains to be seen what impact the most recent report from the Child Safeguarding Practice Review Panel (2022) will have on the way multi-agency reviews are undertaken. The report seeks to share the learning from Arthur and Star and rightly focuses on systemic learning for the safeguarding system, recognising that the experiences of those children whilst tragic, were not unusual. However, a focus on systems, processes, policies, and procedures does not make a demonstrable difference to safeguarding practice in the longer term (Safer Safeguarding Group, 2015). There is a need to consider what additional factors are impacting on the way practitioners think and behave in relation to their safeguarding work if we are to prevent future incidents from occurring.

Practitioner 'burnout' is an individual factor which should be considered as a safeguarding concern as it poses a significant risk to the practitioner's ability to assess and intervene appropriately. When practitioners are stressed, there is the potential that they feel demotivated and develop compassion fatigue – where risks are normalised and not responded to appropriately – and there may be desensitisation of the workforce. In this scenario, practitioners are in danger of screening out the subtleties of risk assessment and analysis, crucial to safeguarding, when they are physically and emotionally exhausted. Action plans can easily become task orientated with little space for reflection or critical thinking.

Learning from Arthur and Star, the report of the Child Safeguarding Practice Review (2022) calls for leaders to take responsibility for creating working conditions that support practitioners to engage with complex work. There is a need to ensure clarity of vision; responsibilities, and resource; robust governance and a culture of learning, improvement, and challenge. There should be clear management oversight of complex safeguarding work, supported by reflective supervision for practitioners. In other words, positive safeguarding practice goes beyond training health and social care practitioners about the legal frameworks and subject matter. It is about creating a working environment where practitioners feel psychologically safe, have the right skills and competence, and have access to appropriate time and resources to perform to their best.

## The child's voice

Lundy (2007) created a model that identifies four distinct factors that should be considered when considering the extent to which a child's participation right can be realised (see Figure 10.2 below). The framework is a helpful model to apply to any investigative process involving children and young people. It ensures that the child's voice is central to the investigation and extends the concept of participation beyond a child's spoken word. When the principle of participation and involvement is understood as a human right, the need to listen to the child's voice in health and social care practice investigations is undeniable.

The four factors of Lundy's participation model are space, voice, audience, and influence. The factors ensure the thread of a child's participation right runs throughout a serious incident investigation. The factors guide investigators to recognise the context (space) and to understand the child's individual experience (voice), so it can be presented to the safeguarding partnership (audience) with a view to learning lessons and changing practice (influence).

Space, according to Lundy, is the opportunity for involvement, where children can express themselves freely and be protected. In order to be able to express a view, children must feel safe and free from influence or any fear of reprisal. They should also be supported to express a view in whatever way they are able. This requires practitioners to tune in to all forms of communication displayed by children and young people, including the need to interpret behaviours as an expression of

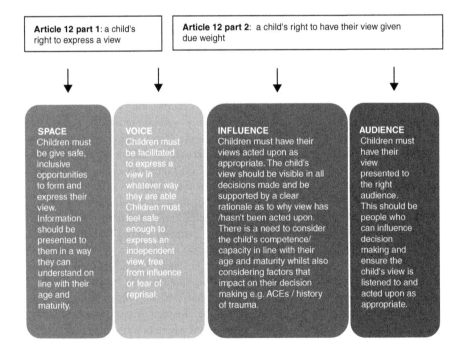

*Figure 10.2* Lundy's Model of Participation

voice. This is especially important when practitioners are working with very young children, children with special educational needs and disabilities (SEND), children with poor mental health, and those for whom English is a second language.

Space can be understood in relation to geography and time, and so provides the social context for any multi-agency review. Geography considers safeguarding thresholds of harm as they are applied at local level, but they must be understood within the political context at a given point in time so the impact on voice, audience, and influence can be recognised.

## Vulnerability

Harrison (2008) describes vulnerability as the 'susceptibility to the unchosen'. Whether or not children are able to participate in their own lives and engage in informed and conscious decision making determines how susceptible they are to the unchosen (Harrison, 2008). Understood in these terms, children are not vulnerable members of society by virtue of age alone. Vulnerability is not associated with age or maturity but is to do with choice, an ability to participate in decision making and exercise agency. Children who can make a choice are therefore less vulnerable as members of society, irrespective of their age or maturity. Choice is created through space where children can express themselves freely, find their voice, and, if presented to the right audience, influence their own safety and wellbeing. A child's right to participate (UNICEF, 1989) is therefore a core principle of safeguarding and child protection. Serious incident investigations involving children should always be conducted in a manner that is sensitive to both the child (if the review does not involve a death) and the family of the child concerned, and also those who have been directly involved with the family.

## Summary

Thresholds for concern and the way in which serious incidents involving children and young people are conducted has evolved considerably in recent years. Child protection in England comprises a complex multi-agency system with many different agencies, organisations, and individuals playing a part. Reflecting on how well that system operates to protect and safeguard children depends on high-quality investigations when a child is seriously harmed or dies and taking the learning from tragic events to better improve services.

The National Independent Inquiry into Child Sexual Abuse regarding the historical abuse of children in care was published in October 2022 comprising 19 reports on 15 investigations. It remains to be seen if this profile and scale of investigation leads to better child protection services and, ultimately, safer care for children and fewer deaths or other serious incidents.

## References

Butler-Sloss, E. (1987). *Report of the Inquiry into Child Abuse in Cleveland.* London: HMSO.

Child Safeguarding Practice Review Panel. (2022). *Child Protection in England: National Review into the Murders of Arthur Labinjo-Hughes and Star Hobson.* Available from: www.gov.uk/government/publications/national-review-into-the-murders-of-arthur-labinjo-hughes-and-star-hobson

Children's Safeguarding and Assurance Partnership. (2021). *Working Well with Children and Families in Lancashire.* Available from: www.lancashiresafeguarding.org.uk/media/19299/wwwcf-part-1-and-2-final.pdf#:~:text=Working%20Together%20%282018%29%20is%20the%20statutory%20guidance%20published,developed%20in%20line%20with%20the%20Working%20Together%20principles.

Department for Education. (2013). *Working Together to Safeguard Children, a guide to inter-agency working to safeguard and promote the welfare of children.* London: HM Government.

Department for Education. (2015). *Working Together to Safeguard Children, a guide to inter-agency working to safeguard and promote the welfare of children.* London: HMSO.

Department for Education. (2018). *Working Together to Safeguard Children, a guide to inter-agency working to safeguard and promote the welfare of children.* London: HMSO.

Department for Education (England). (2016). *Wood Report: Review of the Role and Functions of Local Safeguarding Children Boards.* London: HMSO.

Department for Education. (2020). *Complexity and challenge: A triennial analysis of SCRs 2014–2017. Final report.* London: Department for Education.

Department of Children, Equality, Disability, Inclusion and Youth. (2019), National Framework for Children and Young People's Participation in Decision Making, Government of Ireland. Available from: https://hubnanog.ie/participation-framework

Department of Health. (2000). *Lost in Care: Report of the tribunal of inquiry into the abuse of children in care in the former county council areas of Gwynedd and Clwyd since 1974.* London: HMSO.

Derbyshire Safeguarding Children Board. (2018). *An assurance report reflecting on the current multi-agency safeguarding arrangements within Derbyshire, with reference to Aston Hall Hospital.* Available from: www.ddscp.org.uk/media/derby-scb/content-assets/documents/serious-case-reviews/aston-hall-assurance-report-25-july-2018.pdf

Featherstone, B., Gupta, A., Morris, K., & White, S. (2018) *Protecting Children – A Social Model: Critique of Current Policy and Practice in Child Protection.* Bristol: Policy Press.

Freeman, M, (1996). Children's education; A test case for best interests and autonomy. In *Listening to Children in Education.* Routledge.

Gallacher. L.-A., & Gallagher. M. (2008). Methodological immaturity in childhood research? Thinking through 'participatory methods'. *Childhood*, 15(4), 499–516.

Haringey Safeguarding Children Board. (2008), Ser*ious Case Review 'Child A'.* London: Department for Education.

Harrison, P. (2008). Corporeal remains: Vulnerability, proximity, and living-on after the end of the world. *Environment and Planning A: Economy and Space*, 40(2), 423–445.

HM Treasury. (2003). Every Child Matters. London: HMSO.

HM Government. (2023). Serious Incident Notifications (Financial Year 2021–2022). Available from: https://explore-education-statistics.service.gov.uk/find-statistics/serious-incident-notifications/2021-22

Jay, A., Evans, M., Frank, I., & Sharpling, D. (2022). *The Report of the Independent Inquiry into Child Sexual Abuse.* Available from: www.iicsa.org.uk/reports-recommendations/publications/inquiry/final-report.html

King, A. (2007). The sociology of sociology. *Philosophy of the Social Sciences*, 37, 501–522.

Kingston, P., Eost-Telling, C., & Taylor, L. (2018). *Comparing safeguarding review methodologies.* Available from: www.lancashiresafeguarding.org.uk/media/1110/FINAL-Report-Review-of-safeguarding-methodologies.pdf

Laming, Lord. (2003). *The Victoria Climbié Inquiry.* Norwich: HMSO.

Leonard, M. (2016) *The Sociology of Children, Childhood and Generation.* London: Sage.

London Borough of Brent. (1985). *A Child in Trust: The Report of the Panel of Inquiry into the Circumstances Surrounding the Death of Jasmine Beckford.* London Borough of Brent.

Lundy, L, (2007). 'Voice' is not enough: Conceptualising Article 12 of the United Nations Convention on the Rights of the Child. *British Educational Research Journal,* 33(6), 927–942.

Munro, E. (2011). *Munro Review of Child Protection: Final report – a child centred system,* London: Department for Education.

National Child Mortality Database. (2022). *Sudden and Unexpected Deaths in Infancy and Childhood.* Available from: www.ncmd.info/publications/sudden-unexpected-death-infant-child

National Confidential Inquiry in Suicide and Safety in Mental Health. (2023). Available from: https://sites.manchester.ac.uk/ncish/reports/suicide-by-children-and-young-people

Page, R. (2015). *Clear Blue Water: The Conservative Party and the Welfare State Since 1940.* Bristol: Policy Press.

Prout, A., & James, A. (1997). A new paradigm for the sociology of childhood. In A. James and A. Prout (eds), *Constructing and Reconstructing Childhood: Contemporary Issues in the Sociological Study of Childhood* (2nd ed.). London: Falmer Press.

Safer Safeguarding Group. (2015). *Developing a Responsive Safety Culture in Child Protection Services.* Available from: www.safersafeguardinggroup.amfnet.co.uk

UNICEF. (1989). United Nations Convention on the Rights of the Child (1989). Available from: www.unicef.org.uk/what-we-do/un-convention-child-rights

World Health Organization (WHO). (2019). *Suicide in the World: Global Health Estimates.* WHO. Available from: https://apps.who.int/iris/bitstream/handle/10665/326948/WHO-MSD-MER-19.3-eng.pdf

# 11 Investigations in the custodial setting – practical advice

*David Durrant*

## Introduction

This chapter provides insight and practical advice for the independent investigator who is required to conduct an inquiry within the health sector of a prison. All government guidance described elsewhere within this text applies, along with individual secure service/prison protocols and procedures. The information is drawn from custodial settings, with the focus largely on the prison setting with transferability to other settings such as forensic mental health settings.

## Understanding the custodial setting

A good starting point for any investigation in a prison is to understand the function of the establishment. This can vary in terms of the level of security and categorisation of those held there. For example, an investigation that takes place in a High Security prison will be very different to one in open conditions. The structure of prisons for men is also significantly different to those for women (Kreager et al., 2021). Lastly, you will want to know whether the establishment receives prisoners directly from the courts, as there is likely to be a higher prevalence of unmet medical needs and support required around unstable substance misuse.

Prisons have a clear hierarchy and rank structure (Bennett, 2019), and each establishment will have a governing governor and deputy governor. Prisons are then divided into functions, such as security, residential services, offender management, reducing reoffending, and safer custody. Each will have a governor grade leading them, supported by custodial managers (the highest rank in uniform), supervisory officers, and prison officers. Additionally, operations support grade staff (OSGs) often deliver services in areas such as the main gate and visits, and several different grades of non-operational support staff and managers support delivery. On any given day, there will be a duty governor and orderly officer, who are collectively responsible for the regime and stability of the prison, as well as any initial incident management. There will be a governor grade (often the deputy governor) who oversees healthcare delivery from the prison perspective.

You can expect to encounter cultural, resource, and terminology differences between health environments and prisons, and this chapter will reflect some of these differences.

DOI: 10.4324/9781003286240-15

## Practical considerations and navigating the system

There will be numerous and differing constraints when undertaking interviews and investigations in a prison (Aitkin, 2022). If the investigator is independent of the organisation, they should be allocated a member of staff from within the establishment – for example, the healthcare manager – as they will be aware of key personnel and relevant policies/procedures to liaise with key individuals to manage the practicalities of the task and to reinforce the need for your involvement. Your liaison contact can undertake practical tasks, such as arranging visits, as well as providing information about the prison, its regime, and what to expect. Most importantly, your liaison contact will have keys and so can facilitate your movement around the establishment.

When you arrive at the prison, ensure you have photographic identification with you (e.g. a driving licence) as you will be denied access without this. Also expect that any items being brought into the prison will be searched.

If you are undertaking interviews within the prison, be mindful that many items are prohibited in accordance with security regulations. This means you cannot take mobile phones, recording devices or laptops in with you. Ask your liaison contact to check with the security department about what you can bring into an official visit. Smaller items, such as mobile phones, can be left at the gate in lockers, but not all establishments will have storage for larger items. The security department can be approached to authorise some items, although all establishments will have their own devices for recording interviews, vital if verbatim transcripts are required.

Your access to staff and prisoners will be constrained by the regime (i.e. what happens when in a prison). This will determine how long you have for interviews unless arrangements have been made to cover the member of staff's duties, and there is likely to be limited flexibility about when prisoners are available to you. The choice of where to interview is an important one. Some prisons have facilities outside their perimeter which might be available for staff interviews. This has the advantage of allowing you to use your own laptop or recording devices. In the case of prisoners, all establishments will have facilities for official visits to take place which guarantees you an element of privacy. Further advice is available in PSI 16/2011 Managing prison visits (www.gov.uk).

Alternatives may be rooms in the healthcare unit/wing or in and around the prison's wings. Noise may be an issue, but this may prove a useful approach if you aim to hold a series of short interviews with prisoners from the same location, in a morning or afternoon. You will need to give prisoners notice and gain their consent if you wish to interview them, but they are under no obligation to cooperate. One option is to write, but you are likely to get better outcomes if you can arrange for someone in the prison, ideally your liaison person and preferably someone that a prisoner might know, to explain the purpose of the interview and why they have a contribution to make to the investigation.

It is important that you consider any vulnerabilities associated with a prisoner before meeting them, such as mental or physical health conditions or known learning disabilities, particularly if they are supported through the Assessment, Care in Custody, Teamwork process (ACCT) (PS1 64/2011). It is your responsibility to inform staff of any concerns that you have about the prisoner as a result of your conversation with them, report these immediately after the interview, and provide a written account of concerns.

Ideally, it is helpful to visit the area where an incident took place or the concern arose from. This can help to put things into some context, as well as providing an opportunity for you to get a sense of the dynamics between different groups of staff and their relationships with prisoners as these can be complex within custodial environments (Johansson & Holmes, 2023).

## The politics of your investigation

It is important that your liaison contact ensures that a senior member of prison management is aware of your investigation. There are several reasons for this. First, if an incident has taken place that is sufficiently serious to warrant your investigation, then it is certainly a matter that the prison should be aware of (HMPS, 2014). Second, the governor retains a duty of care to both staff and prisoners; anything that could impact on this, or the dynamics of the establishment, will be a consideration.

Lastly, industrial relations can be complex in prisons (Bennett et al., 2023). Senior managers will need to know if your investigation points to concerns about prison staff. They will certainly want to know if directly employed staff are to be interviewed and to ensure that representation is available and the right processes followed. Consideration needs to be given to whether your investigation stands alone or is a part of a wider suite of enquiries. In complex cases, there may be several organisations undertaking investigations that relate to a specific incident, such as the police and Prison and Probation Ombudsman. In such cases, be aware that any police investigation will always be given primacy (HMPS, 2003, updated 2005). Sensitivity will need to be exercised if there is any investigation taking place suggesting wrongdoing by prison staff.

It is advisable to assess the relationship between health and the wider prison staff (Woodall & Freeman, 2021). There may well be strong bonds because of close working relationships between health and prison staff; if you are undertaking a disciplinary investigation into health staff, be alert to this potential as it may have implications for the levels of cooperation that you receive should you need to interview prison staff (see Chapter 1).

## Sources of information

The following may be useful sources of information when undertaking your investigation. Some will require additional permissions or data-sharing agreements to be in place.

HM Inspectorate of Prisons and the reports of the relevant Independent Mentoring Board can both provide useful information about the establishment and highlight any concerns that these bodies have:

- HM Inspectorate of Prisons – https://hmiprisons.justiceinspectorates.gov.uk
- Independent Monitoring Boards – imb.org.uk

Information about individual prisoners can come from a variety of sources. These include:

- SystmOne for health information.
- Nomis for sentencing details and case notes from staff working with the prisoner.
- OASys for the current assessment of risk of harm and reoffending.
- ACCT documents provide a record of support to a prisoner assessed as vulnerable to self-harming.
- Security information: This is more difficult to access, but a redacted summary of appropriate information may be available in certain circumstances when relevant to the investigation.
- Incidents: Duty governor and orderly officer logs will reference anything operational that caused concern on a given day. More serious incidents will have logs attached to them.
- Complaints: Specific complaints by prisoners about health are likely to have been made through the health provider's own complaints process, and they should hold a log of these. Complaints about most aspects of prison life will be logged by the prison's business hub which will also have copies of the responses sent out.

Information about how prison-commissioned investigations should be undertaken can be found in Prison Service Order 1300 and PSI 15/2014 Investigating incidents of serious self-harm or assault: PSI 15/2014 (www.gov.uk).

**Conclusion**

Investigations in prisons and other secure settings can be complex. You are very much a guest in someone else's territory, with all the challenges that this can bring. There can be a sense of dependency in that you will rely on others to organise and get things done to assist you. However, there are things that you can do to ensure that interviews run smoothly and that you maximise the likelihood of obtaining the information needed to complete the investigation that you have been commissioned to undertake.

**References**

Aitkin, D. (2022). Investigating prison suicides: The politics of independent oversight. *Punishment & Society*, 24(3), 477–497.

Bennett, J. (2019). Reform, resistance and managerial clawback: The evolution of 'reform prisons' in England. *The Howard Journal*, 58(1), 45–64.

Bennett, J., Crewe, B., & Wahidin, A. (2023). *Understanding Prison Staff*. United Kingdom: Willan.

HM Prison Service. (2003, updated 2005). *Police investigations*. Prison Service Order 1300. Available from: https://insidetime.org/wp-content/uploads/2021/12/PSO_1300_investigations.pdf

HM Prison Service. (2014). Investigations and Learning Following Incidents of Serious Self-Harm or Serious Assaults. PSI 15/2014 (Revision). London: HMSO.

Johansson, J. A., & Holmes. D. (2023). Poststructuralism and the construction of subjectivities in forensic mental health: Opportunities for resistance. *Nursing Philosophy*, e12440.

Kreager, D. A., Young, J. T. N., Haynie, D. L., Schaefer, D. R., Bouchard, M., & Davidson, K. M. (2021). In the eye of the beholder: Meaning and structure of informal status in women's and men's prisons. *Criminology*, 59, 42–72.

Woodall, J., & Freeman, C. (2021). Developing health and wellbeing in prisons: An analysis of prison inspection reports in Scotland. *BMC Health Services Research*, 21(1), 314–319, Article 314.

# 12 Investigating within the military context

*James Clapson*

This chapter examines and explores some of the direct implications, considerations, and more appropriate methods (or abilities) of investigating serious incidents within military and hostile or complex environments around the world. Whilst there are many features and conditions that are clearly unique to certain specific geographical environments and conflicts (and therefore either the sole or at least main contributing factors to the types of events and circumstances experienced there), there is still a lot to be gained by viewing the prevalent nature of these environments through the prism of comparison, context, and pattern analysis.

## Complex environments

Investigating serious incidents within certain complex locations such as warzones or hostile environments, usually involves navigating significant constraints and dangers to the individual investigators involved, a practice that can pose an immediate and serious risk to the general safety and/or wellbeing of those exposed to the distinct pressures of these surroundings. Investigators can also be left with lasting distress from their overall experiences there, or from the impact of any specific traumatic event that they either witnessed or investigated, such as delving into the aftermath of systematic violence, extreme human rights violations, or the collection of testimony from victims and survivors. The impact of this exposure can also vary, sometimes through more obvious and rapid-onset emotional trauma, but equally often via a gradual manifestation of symptoms over time – warnings that routinely remain unrecognised, or, more worryingly, are routinely ignored. The effects of long-term suppression can also deepen the effects on the individual and, ultimately, endanger the wider investigative team involved.

Investigations that occur within these environments can also be met by numerous substantial and unconventional hurdles that routinely catch many investigative teams off-guard due to their apparently unexpected nature, alongside the potential degree of complexity involved. But more often than not, these separate and distinct issues can all essentially be traced back to a single point of origin: local corruption. This can be strictly limited to the immediate area of a remote investigation but can equally involve more senior representatives of the regional government, military, and security forces of the nation(s) involved. Environments of this type are also likely to be

DOI: 10.4324/9781003286240-16

deeply troubled by diminished levels of law and order, acute violence, widespread economic hardship, and instability, which present higher degrees of risk to outsiders.

**Threat levels**

The circumstances, incidents and general behaviours that are typically experienced within most military and hostile or complex environments can more easily be recognised and appreciated when viewed as associated but distinct escalations of an inherent risk matrix. These situations exist within states of extreme abnormality, with diverging threats and complications that can often appear to coexist inconspicuously yet retain intrinsic exponential potentials to rapidly worsen without warning. These attributes often also grow or wane in proportion to each other, especially when outside influences combine around them to intensify the wider situation or aggravate local violence, which often results in an emphasis on overtly negative provocations or traits whilst marginalising the more positive and potentially stabilising forces. The early adoption of such a matrix can also be used to better differentiate and demonstrate whenever a previously prevalent trait has become sufficiently diminished (in relation to a newly dominant trait or competitor) that it has now shifted from being a central force to a peripheral one. These escalations are often generalised and typically referred to by individuals operating within hostile environments as incremental 'threat levels'. This term can be used to help better identify potential intensifications in behaviour or events either across isolated or unique unilateral environments (Figure 12.1) or multilaterally, across recurring environments (Figure 12.2).

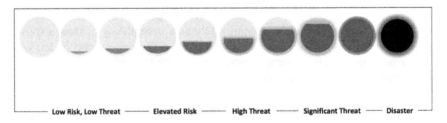

Low Risk, Low Threat ——— Elevated Risk ——— High Threat ——— Significant Threat ——— Disaster

*Figure 12.1* Threat levels within isolated or unique environments

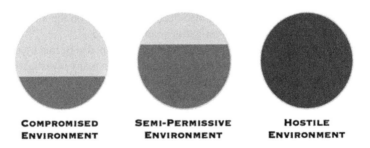

COMPROMISED ENVIRONMENT       SEMI-PERMISSIVE ENVIRONMENT       HOSTILE ENVIRONMENT

*Figure 12.2* Threat levels within or multilaterally across recurring environments

## Types of complex environment

When viewing complex locations such as warzones or hostile environments, it is always useful to first clarify the terminology and descriptions being used to characterise and define them, as this can often provide you with the ability to extrapolate from previous experiences within comparable geographical regions, circumstances, or time periods, such as military conflicts or events involving any widespread hostility, political and civil unrest, insurrection, genocide, humanitarian crises, religious extremism, or ethnic clashes. The most common of these can more accurately be broken down and separated into one of the three following environments (BBC, 2021):

### *'Compromised environments'*

A country or region in which there are well-established perceptions of public sector corruption, extortion, abuse of authority for private gain, and any diplomatic, legal, or economic pressure being brought to bear on individuals by regional or other actors (including the host nation).

### *'Semi-permissive environments'*

A specific environment in which the local national or international security forces operating within can expect to experience variable degrees of obstruction, interference, and resistance, alongside challenges to their authority. The local security situation will likely be volatile and unstable, with restrictions placed on the local movement and international travel of civilians and foreign nationals created by an inability of the host nation to fully impose law and order.

### *'Hostile environments'*

A hostile environment is defined as a country or region that is subject to any war, insurrection, civil unrest, or terrorism, or is facing extreme levels of crime, banditry, lawlessness, or public disorder; typically, a complex or hazardous environment, characterised by its high risk and danger, often remote or difficult to access, with extreme climatic conditions or terrain and natural disasters, such as volcanoes, earthquakes, tsunamis, etc. (BBC, 2021).

## Military environments

Whilst most military environments remain largely distinctive, they all fundamentally exist to conduct warfare against an enemy force that has been determined by an opposing authority. War is timeless; warfare is not. The former describes an activity, one that is bloody, violent, and political, that remains the same in the twenty-first century as it was in the twentieth, or even the fifth. The latter describes how war is conducted or has evolved as a result of improved technologies, geopolitics, ideology, culture, regime changes, and other factors (McFate, 2014).

Most military environments also exist within their own 'bubble', one that is largely unaffected by outside influences and external forces. They can include all manner of physical dangers and genuine risk, and are, by their very nature, *states of emergency*. As such, they are intensely abnormal circumstances that do not easily conform to modern social conventions, ideals, policies, or internationally enforced regulations (Groeben, 2014). Investigators with limited experience of military environments or conflict must also remain aware that any participants that are directly involved within these hostilities, such as combatants and local national militia forces, can often view their particular conflict as an exception to the rules, isolated from other contemporary conflicts, imperative and therefore unlike any other comparable conflicts from the past (unless it suits their particular narrative). This 'tunnel vision' can lead to a collective mentality amongst certain groups where they may start to believe that the *end* justifies any *means*, or, worse, that there is no such thing as 'non-combatants' in their particular area of influence. Whenever you deploy as an investigator to an environment such as this, take every opportunity to err on the side of caution and, if in doubt, move to safety.

Six good rules are:

1. **Atmospherics** – learn to distinguish any *absence of the normal* or *presence of the abnormal*.
2. **Learn to recognise hostility quickly** – there is a huge difference between *irritation* and *anger*.
3. **Learn how to identify potential threats** – lingering stares, being followed, concealed actions.
4. **Avoid routines** – do not become complacent, *avoid being predictable*, change routes often.
5. **Always have somewhere to go** – know your surroundings, visualise your escape routes, know where there are *genuine places of safety* and identify *security forces that can protect you*.
6. **Never second-guess yourself** – *trust your instincts and follow your thought process through*. If something doesn't feel right, do not wait: act on the assumption that something is wrong.

### Real environments with real risks

It remains vitally important to fully understand and appreciate the many dangers that could affect your personal travel towards and away from such environments, as well during your time there. It is highly likely that your investigation has been prompted by a failure of the regional authority that is typically responsible for maintaining effective state security and functional law and order in the area. Under these circumstances, the actual purpose of a serious investigation and its anticipated outcome (to obtain facts and gather evidence regarding a wrongdoing of substantial note) could be in diametric opposition to what the host nation wants to see. Depending on the seriousness of the investigation or the potential identities of those involved, it might be something that the host nation also aims to

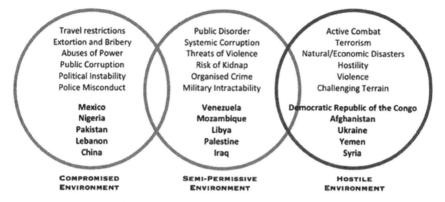

*Figure 12.3* Identified environments with associated risks

see fail, either prior to the arrival of any investigation team or during their actual investigation. As shown in Figure 12.3, these environments are very real, exist in large numbers, and present a great amount of personal risk to investigators via a combination of both unique and universal dangers. When viewed simultaneously, as escalations built upon existing threats (and not just as separate or distinct entities), you can then begin to appreciate that most hostile environments retain both the accumulated features of semi-permissive and compromised environments, as well as the apparent mechanisms behind the intensification of their rising levels of violence and hostility.

## Incidents in complex environments

When conducting any serious investigation within a specific complex environment, you must first acknowledge that the many different behaviours and circumstances occurring within it are ultimately all connected to various degrees, and together form part of a larger abnormal sequence of events that subsequently will not conform to any normal expectations of conduct or conventions you may have. This relates to the type of assistance or reception you might expect, as well as the types of serious incident you can expect to encounter. Local populations may also hold zealously different personal beliefs from you and even maintain value systems that you might find distressing; such as holding a much lower regard for human life than you are typically accustomed to, or maintaining different perceptions of decency in relation to the handling of the bodies of any victims you encounter. As such, it remains vital to accept and understand not only that could you be investigating an atypical serious incident in an abnormal environment, but that your actual conduct of such an investigation will likely also be an abnormal and uncomfortable experience for you as an investigator as well. This could also present itself in a gradual and unexpected way as well, with additional affronts manifesting, either in the form of increasingly limited or complicated access to incident sites developing due to arbitrary security restrictions, or even the conduct and often aggressively vocal opinions of those around you whilst on-site. The main types of investigations you can expect to experience and conduct within complex environments are:

- human rights violations, war crimes, genocide
- air crash Investigations
- outbreaks of disease and epidemics
- election monitoring
- weapon inspection programmes
- kidnap and ransom investigations
- international trade and organised crime investigations
- transnational drug enforcement programmes
- international anti-corruption initiatives
- child exploitation and obscenity investigations
- economic and natural disasters.

### Preparations for complex environments

When starting to prepare for any travel to a complex or military environment, it is important to recognise that the risks do not just begin on your arrival there. *Failing to prepare* for any activity of this nature and scale properly, and promptly, is *preparing to fail*, a saying generally attributed to Benjamin Franklin (1706–1790). Depending on the magnitude of the conflict involved, the number (and identity) of countries with overt or covert interests operating there, the significance of the military forces in play and the level of global media interest in that environment, you could find that both you and your investigation have rapidly become of discernible interest to certain groups and media organisations that might try to contact you before you have prepared yourself for such an encounter. Also, some of the countries you can expect to travel to will often have overly complicated and burdensome administrative processes for obtaining visas and meeting travel requirements. You should also take the time to contact relevant agencies and international organisations such as the World Health Organization, United Nations, and the UK Foreign, Commonwealth and Development Office for updated advice on travel restrictions or route suggestions, and consider your personal welfare and medical needs whilst travelling. Ensure the following are addressed:

- *All* travel requirements have been assessed and planned out.
- *All* logistical requirements have been considered and met.
- *All* emergency requirements have been thought of and integrated.
- *Your* personal protection requirements have been incorporated.
- *Your* specific welfare requirements have been accounted for.
- *Your* emergency contacts have been developed and loaded into phones.
- *Minimum research* – locations, conditions, cultural practices, customs.

### Travelling to complex environments

When investigating an incident with significant repercussions (or as part of a legal mechanism that could be used to bring criminals to justice), it is of vital importance that your entry into any location is safe, legal, and recorded. Outside of the more obvious means of travel available (planes, ship, rail, etc.), there are several specific motivations that can mandate the presence of external or international investigators, and require them to travel into complex or hostile environments that can also be viewed as means or, more exactly, 'methods' of travel.

The foremost methods are as follows:

- external military interventions and peacekeeping mission deployments
- an official/unofficial request for an investigative team by a host nation
- internationally mandated disaster recovery teams
- international reconstruction missions deployed to failing and fragile states
- international agencies and non-governmental organisation deployments
- independent investigations authorised through exceptional circumstances.

Any unauthorised or illegal travel where the arrival of international visitors is undertaken without the approval of a host nation (known as *non-permissive entry* into an environment) can rapidly antagonise any surrounding populations and attract regional animosity, or slowly influence and even aggravate a compromised environment into becoming increasingly more hostile and vastly less permissive over time, or even trigger this conversion instantaneously.

### Deployments in complex environments

When conducting investigations within complex or hostile environments, several key stages must be addressed separately and with enough attention that each point can be planned appropriately in sufficient detail. This process must take into account the risk levels (Figure 12.4).

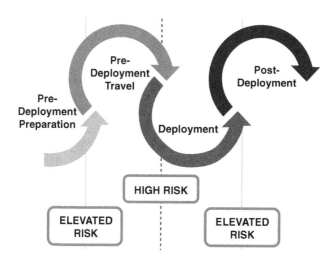

*Figure 12.4* Risk levels across key stages of the investigation

## The four phases of deployment

When assessing the specific and overall requirements for any serious investigation, regardless of the nature and scale of the circumstances and events involved, it is always a good idea to view the process objectively and break it down into four simple but comprehensive sections. This allows you to cover the basics without becoming overwhelmed by any emerging events.

### *Pre-deployment preparation*

1. **Personal preparation** – individual supplies for welfare, medical, life support, and support.
2. **Arrangements** – notifications of travel plans to relevant parties, itinerary preparation.
3. **Travel Plans** – arrangements for domestic and international travel, and host nation travel.
4. **Emergency plans** – emergency return travel, safe havens, alternative travel/escape routes.

### *Pre-deployment travel*

1. **Travel** – personal safety, wellbeing, self-awareness, sleep maintenance, communications.
2. **Arrival** – notify support team, acclimatise, observe, maintain awareness, always alert.
3. **Base of operations** – a place of safety, secured from external actors, safe from theft and harm.
4. **Personal safety** – emergency preparations, protection, contingency planning, escape plans.

### *Deployment*

1. **Familiarisation** – local and regional familiarisation (routes and people), patterns of life.
2. **Situational awareness** – geography, circumstances, history, context, standards, exceptions.
3. **Incident location** – routes to and from incident site and base of operations, scene safety.
4. **Preliminary investigation** – initial enquiries, observations, prioritisation, patterns of life.
5. **Safety on location** – emergency actions, preparations, safe havens, security, escape routes.
6. **Evidence collection** – evidence requirements, relevance, security, chain of custody.
7. **Full investigation** – timeline construction, observations, evidence, investigation objectives.

8. **Conclusions** – immediate conclusions, recommendations, concerns, considerations, notes.
9. **Departure** – arrangements for return travel from host nation (international and domestic).

### Post-deployment

1. **Return travel** – personal safety and wellbeing, self-awareness, alertness, communications.
2. **Report completion** – compile full report and only officially distribute from a place of safety.
3. **Post-deployment administration** – equipment maintenance, welfare and health checks.
4. **Decompression** – establish best sleep pattern quickly, communicate, psychological support.

## Considerations in complex environments

Movement between different cultures and countries can appear seamless to an investigator, and they might often feel that their arrival has barely been noticed, but there are a host of complications that foreign influences (or the arrival of outsiders in a closed environment) can generate. Investigators must remain acutely aware of the impact that both their identity and their potential ignorance of local customs might have on their immediate surroundings. Their presence might also become upsetting or offensive to local communities that are unfamiliar with foreign cultures and foreigners, and cultural oversights or associated mistakes can often aggravate an already precarious situation. When deploying to a new environment, take extra time to become more culturally aware, as this could make the difference between completing a successful investigation and being forced to quickly leave an area. The main exceptional and abnormal circumstances to consider when operating within any complex environments are:

- **Danger** – your perception of a hazard or risk might not be the same as nearby local nationals.
- **Changing circumstances** – national events could have an unforeseen impact on your region.
- **Religious events or holy periods** – particular festivals or symbolic events can turn previously friendly local national sentiment into irritation and even direct hostility towards outsiders.
- **International events** – unrecognised foreign events can have hugely significant or symbolic effects on local national populations in your area (e.g. 9/11 and the Middle East).
- **Seasonal changes in unfamiliar climates** – being unprepared for hot or cold climates, or rainy seasons, can create an atmosphere of pity or distaste for you for you amongst local nationals.

- **Cultural clashes** – Ignorance to local customs or dress codes can generate instant hostility.
- **Unfamiliarity with corruption** – being offended or refusing to comply with locally accepted levels of corruption could be seen as offensive to local nationals in your immediate area.

## Summary

As with any investigation, always prioritise your foreground research. Clearly identify the incident in question and its characteristics, and identify the objectives that need to be achieved. Determine the timeframe that is available and identify the resources and support you have in place or will need. Understand the environment that you are deploying to. Become culturally aware and plan ahead. Try to think of every possible scenario that could occur, good or bad, and try to establish a rough idea of what you will do in these situations – where you could go, how you could get there, who might be able to help you. Ensure that you have good equipment and communication strategies ready, then build a contingency plan in case your primary means of communication fail you. Remain calm and motivated, but also remain alert once you deploy. Avoid complacency and never lose your situational awareness.

As discussed, there is a lot more to conducting investigations within complex and military environments than just having good intentions or vast investigative experience. Much more. For those with limited experience of foreign cultures or minimal exposure to violence and hostility, there is still much that can be established within the pre-deployment phase that will enable you to better navigate the challenging circumstances and potential hostility that lies ahead. An open mind, the ability to learn, humility, and an openly receptive stance towards foreign customs and cultural mannerisms will do more to aid you in your task than a lifetime of experience ever could, especially in the face of any local national hostility and resistance. Investigations in these environments may appear to be an impossible task when viewed from only one angle, especially if under pressure, but when seen holistically, you can slowly start to appreciate what might ultimately become possible. With this in mind, there is little that cannot be achieved by the right person in the right place. So, consider these last deliberations, and remember, *everybody has a plan until they get punched in the mouth…*

- You can either do things the right way or the quick way, but these are rarely the same thing.
- Identify what you can and can't do straight away.
- Prioritise what you can do, ignore what you can't, and just work your way through the rest.
- Quickly establish your professional identity.
- You will often find that your early achievements start to have a ripple effect on the things you initially perceived as being unachievable – it could even inspire others to help you with them.

- Trust should always be *earned*, never given freely. Do not blindly trust the first person to help you, but do not ignore friendliness when others are hostile. Invest in these relationships and allow others to earn your genuine trust, whilst you earn theirs. This will be your greatest asset.

## References

BBC. (2021). *Hostile Environments Defined.* British Broadcasting Corporation. Safety Guides. Available from: www.bbc.co.uk/safety/safetyguides/highrisk/hostile-environments

Groeben, C. von der. (2014). *Transnational Conflicts and International Law* (Vol. 3). Books on Demand.

McFate, S. (2017). *The Modern Mercenary: Private Armies and What They Mean for World Order.* Oxford University Press.

# 13 Fitness to practise investigations

*Joanne Keeling*

## Introduction

Within this chapter the purpose and nature of fitness to practise (FtP) will be discussed as it applies to registrants, clinicians, and healthcare professionals and students (hereafter referred to as 'the practitioner'). Examples of regulatory body processes to examine FtP will be provided along with case study examples to illustrate this complex type of investigation.

## Background

All professional regulatory bodies of health professions have a common statutory responsibility to 'protect the public' (Health and Social Care (Safety and Quality) Act 2015). Within this responsibility is the duty to ensure that practitioners instil public confidence in their respective professions, promote the health and wellbeing of individuals, and maintain professional standards. When there are concerns or allegations about the fitness to practise of an individual which may jeopardise this remit, a FtP investigation by the regulatory body may be initiated. The primary purpose of this type of investigation is to decipher whether an individual is or is not fit to practice, or whether they are impaired in some way that renders them unsafe without support or supervision.

Issues that warrant an FtP investigation centre around the lack of health, competence, and/or conduct and character of a practitioner, including that which falls outside the working environment such as criminal convictions and cautions. In each case, the facts of the matter need to be first established and the severity assessed; the potential risk to public health and safety is always of paramount importance.

Any party, including lay people, can report concerns about a practitioner to the relevant regulatory body, and there is extensive guidance on individual regulatory body websites for anyone wishing to do so within each organisation's publicly shared processes. Similarly, there is a professional duty to self-refer to the regulatory body should they be subject to any procedures or concerns that they feel put their fitness to practise into question. If concerns are raised in an employment environment – for example, against a practitioner

DOI: 10.4324/9781003286240-17

by a colleague or manager – it initially falls on the employer to investigate such matters. Usually, this will involve the human resources department and an appointed impartial investigator, and will follow the procedures set out in a contract of employment. An investigatory or disciplinary process may follow, under the auspices of employment law. It is then the decision of an employing organisation about whether the matter warrants reporting to the regulatory body.

However, it does not follow that a regulatory body will issue the same sanctions or decisions as the employing body may have done: a disciplinary procedure by an employer against a practitioner may not warrant any further action under FtP procedures. This is why communication between relevant parties is essential in order to ensure that processes are aligned to ensure expedience and a thorough consideration of the facts.

In recent times, regulatory bodies have reviewed processes to ensure they work together sensibly with employers to embed the principles of 'right touch regulation', which emphasises communication, proportionality, and transparency between relevant parties (Professional Standards Authority for Health and Social Care, 2015).

FtP investigations are often multifaceted in that they invariably involve a complainant, healthcare staff, witnesses involved in the case, and the employer. Cases may also involve a professional union representative and, in the case of registrant practitioners, the regulatory body such as the Health and Care Professions Council (HCPC) for allied health professionals, the General Medical Council (GMC) for doctors, and the Nursing and Midwifery Council (NMC) for nurses, nursing associates, and midwives. In this respect, FtP investigations can be a stressful and worrying time for all involved, and it is important that people feel supported throughout.

Whilst the main purpose of any FtP investigation is to assess the risk and potential or actual harm to the public, it is important that this is balanced by the premise that until procedures have reached a conclusion, everyone has the right to be supported and aware of what support is available. This is particularly pertinent where a practitioner has informed the regulatory body that they have been subject to procedures which could put their fitness to practise in question. This is a responsibility of the practitioner under their professional code and can place the individual in a precarious and what may seem lonely position both with the regulator and their employer (Worsley et al., 2017).

Following an FtP investigation, and in the event that allegations are deemed proven, there are a range of employment and regulatory body sanctions that can be applied both during an investigation and following an investigative outcome, ranging from suspension or interim orders (whilst the facts are determined) to certain restrictions upon practice, disciplinary sanctions, suspension from the professional register, or removal from the professional register completely, leading to dismissal from employment. Thus, the outcome of an FtP investigation is rarely solely a binary decision.

### Case Study 1

Simone (pseudonym) is a 25-year-old registered occupational therapist who one evening is involved in an incident in a nightclub which results in her arrest. She is subsequently taken to the police station and accepts a caution for assault under the advisement of a solicitor. Simone is very upset and informs the police that she is a registrant. The police explain that they have a common law disclosure power (College of Policing, 2016) to inform the regulator directly regarding Simone's caution.

Simone informs her employer of the caution she has received; the employer subsequently suspends Simone from employment pending a disciplinary investigation. Simone's employer discusses with Simone the duty to inform the Health and Care Professions Council of the situation whether or not the disciplinary investigation finds that Simone should be formally disciplined or further sanctioned. With the support of her union representative, Simone telephones the HCPC who make a file note of the referral and ask that Simone keeps in contact with any developments. The HCPC also contact Simone's employer requesting that they be informed of the outcome of the proceedings. After a week, the HCPC contact Simone to let her know that the police have also been in touch with details of the caution. Simone is ultimately given a written warning from her employer. She and her employer both inform the HCPC who then consider the case at the triage stage.

### Case Study 2

Peter (pseudonym) is a registered nurse working on an in-patient area. On an early shift, Peter's ward manager notices that Peter appears lethargic and 'absent-minded' whilst going about his duties. The ward manager speaks with Peter and further notices that Peter smells of stale alcohol. During conversation, Peter discloses that he has been offered help before for a drinking problem 'several times over the past six months' but that he feels that his drinking 'is not a problem' and has no effect on his job. Peter is quite hostile and aggressive when questioned further and offered occupational health support; the ward manager sends him home from duty. Later that day, Peter's colleague reports that there are some anomalies in the drug administration records signed by Peter. Despite Peter signing to confirm medication has been administered, several patients complain that they did not receive their medications that morning, requiring several individual patient assessments to determine if any harm was apparent. An untoward incident is reported, and Peter is informed that he will be suspended from duty pending an investigation. The ward manager seeks advice from the Nursing and Midwifery Council as she feels that Peter has very little insight into the impact of his drinking on his health. She also feels that this is affecting his performance at work and that he poses a significant risk to patients.

**Example of regulatory body FtP procedures/processes**

*Health and Care Professions Council (HCPC)*

The HCPC is responsible for the regulation of 15 health and care professions in the United Kingdom. Generic standards of conduct, performance, and ethics coupled with profession-specific standards of proficiency provide a template of what is expected of registrants. The HCPC offer extensive guidance on their website about raising concerns and give examples of the types of issues that should be referred to them 'regardless of the outcome of any disciplinary, performance or other issue' (HCPC, 2019). The types of cases the HCPC consider are those of misconduct, lack of competence, caution or conviction, and unmanaged mental or physical health condition affecting safe practice. Consideration by the HCPC would normally occur following the outcome of any disciplinary/employment procedures, but it would not necessarily follow that the same outcome would be arrived at by the HCPC and the employer.

First, the HCPC would assess whether the case would be something they would deal with (the 'triage stage') and, if so, proceed to an investigatory stage. The investigation would involve collating information to ascertain the extent of the concerns raised and whether a practitioner's fitness to practise is impaired. This is assessed using the HCPC Threshold Policy for FtP Investigations and the Health Professions Order (2001) which sets out the statutory reasons why a registrant might be impaired to practise. If the HCPC consider the threshold to be met, allegations will be devised and referred to an investigatory committee. At this stage, the committee decides whether there is a case to answer based on the evidence; if there is, the registrant is informed and given 28 days to respond to the allegations. This response is paper based, and the registrant does not appear in person in front of any panel. Once responses have been received from the registrant, the investigating committee panel meets privately and responds in writing. If the panel feel that the case needs further investigation and sanctions are likely to be needed, it refers to legal representation in preparation for a final hearing. At this hearing, the registrant, if found impaired or not fit to practise, receives a sanction ranging from a caution, a conditions of practice order, or being struck from the register. The registrant must appeal to the High Court if he/she considers the sanction unfair or wrong.

*Nursing and Midwifery Council (NMC)*

The NMC is responsible for the regulation of nurses, midwives, and nursing associates in the UK. The Council's main regulatory aim is the protection of the public.

They state that the two aims for fitness to practice are (i) '[a] professional culture that values equality, diversity and inclusion, and prioritises openness and learning in the interests of patient safety' and (ii) '[n]urses, midwives and nursing associates who are fit to practise safely and professionally' (NMC, 2024).

The NMC have 12 principles upon which they make decisions in relation to FtP allegations, and they have produced a 'Fitness to Practice library' on their website. Allegations that the NMC will consider focus upon issues related to misconduct, lack of competence, criminal convictions and cautions, health, lack of knowledge of English, determinations by other health and social care organisations, and incorrect or fraudulent entry on to the professional register.

Similar to the HCPC, the NMC screen cases to assess the level of seriousness and use threshold standards. They decide whether a case warrants an investigation and can impose interim orders, such as suspension from the register, to protect the public whilst the case is progressed. Any resultant hearings are a matter of public record, available on their website, and registrants attend hearings with representation in order to explain their perspective on events.

### Health care professions students/learners/apprentices

Unfortunately, sometimes allegations or concerns are raised about a pre-registration/pre-qualifying healthcare student which may be necessary to progress and deal with under FtP procedures, in order that the public are protected. As the regulatory bodies deal only with registrants, it is the remit of the educational body to investigate such matters and for this reason many higher education institutions (HEIs) have local FtP policies and procedures in place. Clearly, the same level of competence cannot be expected from students as from registrants, as students are learners. However, as students are the registrants of the future, it is important that they are aware of the requirements of being fit to practise and that the protection of the public is paramount.

Sometimes a student may not fully understand what becoming a member of a healthcare profession entails from the outset of their programme of study, so it is essential that introducing students to professional standards, and what this means for practice and conduct as an individual, is introduced very early on and repeated formally at least annually. This could align with the requirement for students to declare annually they are of good character and health as is a condition by some professional bodies of programme validation. There is a wealth of information available for students in terms of what is expected of them as a learner/student healthcare professional, and the NMC, HCPC, and GMC, to name but a few, have published extensive guidance on their respective websites.

In order that students and practice educators know the procedure for reporting fitness to practise issues, it is useful that HEIs have established protocols including templates to be used that are accessible to all, should FtP concerns and allegations be raised about a learner. Any template should include the nature of the allegation, the time(s) and dates of the specific occurrence(s), how the behaviour/actions of the learner are not in keeping with the relevant profession-specific code or expectations, the names of witnesses involved, and contact details. It is also important that practice educators and supervisors in practice have a named contact within the HEI that they can reach to ask for support and guidance.

There is a requirement that students are supported locally if they are subject to concerns about their health, conduct, or level of competence, so HEIs should have a process in place for dealing with such matters: this will be a condition of programme validation. It is the responsibility of the hosting HEI to confirm at the end of a programme of study whether the learner/student is fit to practise, so accurate recording of any incidents is essential.

## Conclusion

Being fit to practise is a fundamental requirement of any healthcare professional or student/learner, and when this is called into question, cases can be complex and stressful for all involved. Thankfully, regulatory bodies and professional bodies now have extensive guidance for registrants, students, employers, and the public. It is the primary purpose of any FtP procedures to ensure that members of the public always remain protected.

## References

College of Policing. (2016). Common Law Police Disclosure. Available from: www.gov.uk/government/publications/common-law-police-disclosure

Health and Care Professions Council. (2019). Fitness to Practise. Available from: www.hcpc-uk.org/concerns/what-we-investigate/fitness-to-practise

Health and Care Professions Council. (2016). *Guidance on Conduct and Ethics for Students*. Available from: www.hcpc-uk.org/globalassets/resources/guidance/guidance-on-conduct-and-ethics-for-students.pdf

Health and Social Care (Safety and Quality) Act 2015. Available from: www.legislation.gov.uk/ukpga/2015/28/contents

The Health Professions Order 2001. Available from: www.legislation.gov.uk/uksi/2002/254/contents/made

Nursing and Midwifery Council. (2024). Fitness to Practise library. Available from: www.nmc.org.uk/ftp-library

Professional Standards Authority for Health and Social Care (2015) Right-touch regulation. Available from: www.professionalstandards.org.uk/what-we-do/improving-regulation/right-touch-regulation

Worsley, A., McLaughlin, K., & Leigh, J. (2017) A subject of concern: The experiences of social workers referred to the Health and Care Professions Council. *The British Journal of Social Work*, 47(8), 2421–2437.

## Useful resources

British Medical Association. (2020). Ethics Toolkit for Medical Students. Available from: www.bma.org.uk/advice-and-support/ethics/medical-students/ethics-toolkit-for-medical-students/medical-students-and-the-gmc

Nursing and Midwifery Council. (2022) Health and Character as a Student. Available from: www.nmc.org.uk/education/becoming-a-nurse-midwife-nursing-associate/guidance-for-students

# 14 Managing organisational dynamics

*Jo Ramsden*

## Introduction

This chapter considers incident investigation within the context of unconscious organisational processes which influence practice. How these practices become routine and unnoticed – only revealed when something goes wrong – highlights the importance of routine structures which allow workers to think.

A worker, new to an NHS Trust, attended a weekly team meeting. She arrived on time and sat in the room waiting for others who all eventually arrived late. There was no agenda, minutes, or previous actions for the meeting and a significant number of people had sent apologies. Given what was unfolding, the worker enquired about the significance of the meeting and how valuable it was in terms of decision making. People seemed surprised she had asked these questions, and no satisfactory answer was given. Later, several people who had attended the meeting came, uninvited and individually, to the new worker's office to explain, confidentially, that the meeting had been very difficult in the past. The meeting had had the capacity to expose some complicated relationships and had left people feeling very uncomfortable. The new worker felt embarrassed that she had exposed these difficulties and, on attending the meeting in the future, never again raised questions or concerns.

Many of us believe that 'work' is a rational pursuit and that the task we are focused on when we are at work is explicit and unchanging. Despite this, we are also aware of the many frustrations, crises, grievances, etc. which litter our days, and which often obstruct our more purposeful endeavours. In the example above, we can see that, in all likelihood, the meeting continued to be ineffective and wasteful in terms of time and resources because of emotional processes which could not be managed. It was easier, and may have felt safer, for the new worker to adapt to the culture and cease to notice how the meeting was no longer serving the purpose for which it was intended but had begun to

DOI: 10.4324/9781003286240-18

operate strangely and in a way that served a different purpose – of avoiding conflict, perhaps. For many of us, these examples may be less obvious than the one above but may, nonetheless, intrude into our consciousness through their ability to interfere with and frustrate what we want and hope to achieve in our working lives:

> Deeply prosaic pre-occupations with bureaucracy and finance mix with critical existential concerns on a daily basis in human services. There are conversations that can never get started because of the language and cultural differences of disciplines, departments and sectors. There are conflicts which never end because of one or another project or clique gets stuck in grievance. There are risks to sanity in attempting to make sense of resource constraints in relation to commissioning demands. There are extreme provocations to the will to live in the neoliberal marketisation of public sector services, with, in some instances, completely unrealistic and deeply punitive inspection frameworks and performance indicators designed to identify successes and failures based on instruments which are inappropriate for human service evaluation. The discontents are legion.
>
> (Barrett, 2020: 113)

All these interferences are likely to emerge from a variety of different sources and, evidently, some of the things that frustrate workers will be necessary for good and safe working (e.g. mandatory training or line management supervision). This chapter, however, is concerned with the influences that problematically disrupt the structures and processes necessary for safe, effective, and person-centred care.

An *open systems model* for understanding human services will be outlined here as a way of helping us to identify these types of influences. How and why they emerge will then be discussed, with reference to the psychodynamic literature on organisational anxiety. This chapter will argue that it is tasks which are unconsciously directed towards the alleviation of organisational stress that disrupt the containing structures of our services, and that these tasks add to the stresses inherent in work which is focused on caring for and managing other human beings. Critically, these unconscious tasks constitute a powerful deviation from person-centred or values-based practice and often result, therefore, in failure and/or harm. Consequently, this chapter will suggest that it is often when something has gone wrong – when there is an incident – that the influence of the unconscious life is noticed.

For many authors who contribute to the psychodynamic literature on organisational dynamics, it is accepted that work in the human services inevitably involves confronting 'powerful and primitive emotional states' (Krantz, 1994: xiv). For these authors, therefore, when we are engaged in our work, we are also pursuing a set of unconscious tasks focused on the alleviation of emotional discomfort (Obholzer & Zagier Roberts, 1994). These tasks – variously referred to in the literature as social defences (Menzies, 1961), anti-task activities (Zagier Roberts, 1994), or operational principles (Barrett, 2020) – may frustrate us as workers, but they may also feel responsible or rational or just 'what we do around here'.

The theme of this chapter will be that, through being unnoticed, unquestioned, and driven by emotion, the unconscious life of a team or system is powerfully able to evade accurate assessment by investigators. Any organisation which has a large collection of investigation reports but which has also failed to learn (i.e. where the reports continue to say the same things) has, arguably, a body of cumulative evidence for disruptive unconscious processes. When we fail to learn and change things effectively, we might assume that either these unconscious processes can't be identified or named (and we are trying to learn the wrong thing) or that an investigation has uncovered the need for change which is so anxiety provoking that change is impossible.

This chapter concludes by making some recommendations for the conditions which need to be in place for effective learning to occur. Fundamentally, these require an appreciation for and an acceptance of the reality of an unconscious life and humility about the fallibility of all of us as workers. The myth of rational expertise and unclouded professional judgement is problematic for human services which seek to build 'real' teams (Lyubovnikova et al., 2015) who manage stress well and work effectively with other people's suffering.

## An 'open systems' approach to understanding organisations

Vega Zagier Roberts (1994) describes an 'open system' as being one which is porous enough to take in what it requires from the environment and robust enough to ensure that the important material remains inside and can be converted into whatever the system requires for its output. This analogy, drawn from nature and from the study of living organisms, is useful for helping us to think about the human services and what they require to function well. Barrett (2020) uses the example of a university which is required to allow a steady stream of learners inside. The containing space inside the university needs to be robust enough to allow those learners to absorb new knowledge and, where relevant, let go of things they may have previously understood. Educators, too, must work across this permeable boundary – contributing to and receiving new knowledge which might be generated outside the university so it may be brought in and used for learning. The output is the student with a degree certificate confirming the level of knowledge they have about the relevant subject.

In her analogy of a university as an open system, Barrett (2020) draws our attention to the factors in this model which shape the output: each university graduate is created, in part, by the requirements of the university (an individual with a degree is the required output), in part by their individual capacity to learn (the nature of the material), but also by the quality of the structures used to manage various boundaries on their learning journey. This boundary management enables 'containment' of the throughput and the effective delivery of a satisfactory output. These boundaries exist at the internal/external and entry/exit margins, but also between different functions or parts (or departments) inside the organisation. When we consider the organisation in this way, we can start to imagine various potential boundary containment failures, all of which would potentially impact on the learning journey for students: warring or competing departments, poorly financed resources, lecturers preoccupied by external or internal events, etc.

This book is concerned with the investigation and learning from serious failures and/or harm. To put this another way, the topic of interest is how to understand it when the required output (a supported human being who is suffering less) is somehow prevented or obstructed. What is of interest and relevance to this chapter, then, is the (often unconscious) factors which interfere with boundary management and prevent us from effectively attending to the task of working with human beings.

## Task

Clarity about the primary task of an organisation facilitates effective containment of its systems and is essential for its survival in relation to demands from outside its system boundary (Barrett, 2020; Miller & Rice, 1967). However, defining a primary task for human services is complex, given the multiple demands placed on them alongside the need to constantly shift in the face of frequent change, reorganisation, and 'transformation'.

Despite this, it is essential for an organisation to achieve clarity in its systems if the working of that organisation is to remain unproblematic. Nowhere is this better illustrated than in the Mid Staffordshire NHS Foundation Trust Public Inquiry in 2013. In his letter to the then secretary of state for health, Robert Francis QC describes a culture of competing and confusing tasks which were pursued by the Trust, and which resulted in serious failings in patient care (Mid Staffordshire NHS Foundation Trust Public Inquiry, 2013). For example, he describes a focus on achieving a foundation trust status and an over-preoccupation with positive information and compliance. In his overarching recommendation (to instil a culture of putting the patient first), he highlights the importance of attending to the boundaries which will enable the required output (good patient care).

Zagier Roberts (1994) suggests that confusion about the primary task within helping institutions and the communities and society that they serve often results in inadequate or vague task definitions. She suggests that this then provides 'little guidance to staff or managers about what they should be doing, or how to do it' (30). In their research examining culture and behaviour in the English NHS system, Dixon Woods and colleagues (2014) found that consistent achievement of high-quality care by committed and professional staff was challenged by 'unclear goals' and 'overlapping priorities' (106).

For Zagier Roberts (1994), the problems with task definition which plague those in the human services often result from confusion between methods and aims, difficulties in prioritising activities and failure to shift gear or change task in relation to changing environments.

**Case example**

An NHS Trust concerned with re-designing clinical governance structures highlighted the importance of learning within the new arrangements they had made. It was hoped that the new focus on learning would reduce high rates of staff sickness, restraint, and serious incidents. The design team agreed that hearing how learning affected the patient journey was key to ensuring that the learning section of the new governance committee meeting was working well and having an impact. Teams were, therefore, put on to a rota to bring a learning story each month. Despite the wealth of positive patient stories which were subsequently brought to the committee, incident rates and staff well-being across the organisation were unaffected. The committee chair took it upon herself to interview managers and lead clinicians to find out more about the stories that were being brought. These interviews revealed that teams were not operating any differently but, that 'finding a learning story' had become a new task which was added to their routine way of working. In addition, it emerged that team leaders were also focused on ensuring that the 'learning story' was positive.

In the example above, we can see how easily a well-intentioned initiative becomes a new primary task. In this example, we might assume that the learning stories were intended to reflect changes to operations, but, in fact, they became a task in themselves. The scrutiny that would have been brought by the committee (whether or not that was their explicit intention) meant that teams alleviated any anxiety by ensuring that the new task was conducted in a way that reflected on them positively.

**Operational principles**

Operational principles may be written down but may also exist unconsciously within an organisation and interfere with efforts to manage boundaries necessary for a desired output. Given that much of the work in the helping institutions is done in teams, there are efforts within the literature to understand how systems begin to be shaped by the needs of people working in groups. Stokes (1994), for example, describes how groups and teams may face a powerful conflict in both wishing to engage in real work (primary task) but also to avoid work focused on the primary task when it's painful (Menzies, 1961) or when group relations make work difficult. When this happens, the unconscious avoidance of pain and conflict can mean that practices emerge which are related to the survival of the group not as defined by those in the external environment (e.g. commissioners) but by the internal needs of the group and their psychological and emotional survival (Stokes, 1994).

Although Lyubovnikova and West (2013) champion the better decision making and effective performance of well-structured, highly functioning teams, they also draw attention to the factors that characterise poorly functioning teams and which underpin failures to achieve many important outcomes for patients. These characteristics include status hierarchies and avoidance of problem identification (Nembhard & Edmondson, 2006); ignoring best practice in the interests of team relationships (Lewis & Tully, 2009); a lack of focus on patient care (Ross et al., 2000); and failure to collaborate with others.

These characteristics might be viewed within our open systems framework as unconscious, anti-task activities which interfere, sometimes catastrophically, with the team's capacity to manage the boundaries necessary for the outcome they are trying to achieve. It is, perhaps, tempting to assume that these anti-task activities – maybe because they are less rational – are easy to identify and remedy. What we should acknowledge, however, is their capacity to powerfully influence and sustain mindless cultures within which poor, sometimes abusive practices can flourish.

I do not for a moment believe that those in responsible positions in the Trust or elsewhere in the healthcare system went about their work knowing that by action or inaction they were contributing to or condoning the continuance of unsafe or poor care of patients. What is likely to be less comfortable for many of those in such posts at the time is the possibility, and sometimes the likelihood, that whatever they believed at the time, they were not being sufficiently sensitive to signs of which they were aware with regard to their implications for patient safety and the delivery of fundamental standards of care (Mid Staffordshire NHS Trust Public Inquiry, 2013).

Arguably, one reason these types of wilfully blind (Heffernan, 2013) cultures exist is because there is a lack of an appreciation for the emotional burden of the work that those in the human services are engaged in. Menzies (1961), for example, highlighted the fear and anxiety that was elicited in nurses in a large teaching hospital in London as they sought to care for patients with a range of physical health problems. In this seminal paper, she describes the range of practices that emerged within the culture of the hospital, all of which were felt to be rational and professionally responsible and all of which were organisationally sanctioned but which, nonetheless, constituted unconscious attempts to manage unspoken anxiety in the workforce at the expense of good patient care.

Barrett (2020) is also at pains to stress how unconscious operational principles may also be unnoticed and unnamed because they are essential – either for avoiding the painful nature of the work or for continued functioning in the face of immense financial or other resource pressures or the mindless demands of accountability. This author stresses the importance of retaining compassion for operational principles which may have constituted the best and most effective forms of power and survival for embattled teams and organisations.

The very nature, therefore, of the types of processes which distort practice and which (according to the open systems model) disrupt effective boundary management are that they are uncomfortable, powerful, and rarely observed or named. Hinshelwood (2002), for example, describes how a primary task to 'help' can be unconsciously and mindlessly distorted into a form of unconscious abuse without structures in place to help notice what is happening.

## Relevance to incident investigations

Given all the above, we might be able to view incident investigations as an activity which studies the 'symptoms' or observable features of these unconscious influences. Practices that fail to serve the human beings we are working with, and which result, therefore, in some form of failure or harm are, in many cases, likely to constitute some form of boundary mismanagement which prevents our open systems from producing the required output of a healthier, better functioning human being. Arguably, an incident investigation is a good opportunity to notice what is happening as the powerful influences which distort patient-focused practices are often hard to name for a variety of reasons. In the example given at the start of this chapter, we can see how it became more important to disrupt or obstruct the meeting than it did to make it work. If we assume this meeting had a clinical function, then the unconscious task of disrupting it starts to work against the interests of service users and their families. What is also important to note about this example are the very powerful influences that started to shape the new worker's ability to feel safe enough to notice and comment upon the anti-task activity around the meeting. Tacitly, she was invited to collude with the anti-task activity and to protect her colleagues from the stress and anxiety involved in grappling with whatever was required to make the meeting work.

It is, perhaps, important to acknowledge that it is partly in response to the recognition of how hard it is to notice powerfully protected anti-task activities that there are efforts to support those who wish to 'blow the whistle' (e.g. Freedom to Speak Up guardians within the NHS; NHS England, 2022). Whilst these efforts are admirable, it does potentially perpetuate a discourse and a media narrative that 'speaking up' about things that are going wrong means, to put it in the simplest terms, good people noticing bad things (maybe enacted by bad people). This can be seen in the BBC *Panorama* documentary on the Edenfield Centre in Prestwich (BBC, 2022). If we contrast this with the example early in this chapter regarding the meeting, we can see that the behaviour of the new staff member which perpetuated the status quo was not the action or inaction of a 'bad' person but was instead the result of powerful layers of influence.

Incident investigators are unlikely to be faced routinely with deeply abusive and abhorrent situations (although, of course, this does happen) and, instead, are more likely to be investigating unfortunate events which happen despite the efforts of committed, passionate, and dedicated workers operating within powerful systems that apply unseen influences on their practice.

### Case example

A care coordinator within the NHS was interviewed following the death by suicide of one of his patients. It was noticed that, on the safety plan completed shortly before the patient died, a number of measures had been cited as ways the patient would keep himself safe. It was evident to the incident reviewer that these measures were likely not to be effective, and it was also notable that the patient had cited using the same safety techniques in the past before previous suicide attempts. The patient's own assessment of himself was in contrast to the risk assessment, completed by the care coordinator, which rated his risk as high. When asked about this discrepancy, the care coordinator talked about how the training he had received on completing safety plans had stressed the importance of this being a patient-led process. The training had led him to believe that the safety plan process was more relevant and important than what was considered by the organisation to be an inadequate risk assessment process. The care coordinator felt nervous about asserting his assessment of the patient's risk given that the patient had so confidently talked about how well he would manage. The care coordinator believed that he would be criticised for not practising in a patient-centred way if he were to declare his concerns.

In the above example, we can see how important issues such as patient choice and person-centred care may have led to unconscious anxiety within the system about practice which might be felt to be overly directive. The safety plan initiative was probably an attempt to manage this anxiety and, in seeking to manage anxiety (rather than to thoughtfully shape practice), inadvertently became what was felt to be the task for this worker, resulting in a blindly patient-led approach. Following the patient (and ignoring his own judgement) became an anti-task activity which served organisational anxiety at the expense of the service user. We could only guess at how difficult it may have been within this culture for the care coordinator to intimate that his patient was not the best judge of his own risk.

This example also helps to illustrate what are some of the defining character-istics of anti-task activity: it is in the nature of unconscious and unexamined 'so-cial defences' (Menzies, 1961) that distress, dissatisfaction, and anxiety within the workforce is increased. In addition, anti-task influences have the capacity to in-crease other, more destructive emotions. Hinshelwood (2002), for example, talks about how staff teams may come to experience hatred or contempt for those they care for as a distortion of their 'frustrated inability to understand what is happening to them' (S20). In other words, when boundaries are mismanaged, and practices emerge which situate workers in more anxious and challenging circumstances, dis-satisfaction and frustration may become problematically and inappropriately fo-cused on patients. The relevance to incident investigations is clear, and we can also see how discourses (and media reports) of 'bad' nurses/social workers/doctors, etc. tend to perpetuate difficulties by ignoring far more important powerful organisa-tional structures and cultures.

For investigators, too, the influences which unconsciously lead to anti-task ac-tivities and practices may affect an ability to notice and to speak. It is possible that investigators, when encountering these influences, may experience them as so overwhelming and significant for the teams that it might feel safer to notice and comment upon something else. Equally, it is possible that the implications of noticing anxiety within the teams are so far-reaching and labyrinthian for the organisation that it is, again, easier to notice something else.

## The conditions for learning well

To summarise, this chapter is concerned with powerful unconscious factors which distort the boundaries necessary for healthy, person-centred human services. We have suggested that these factors tend to remain unnoticed and unspoken, meaning that they are difficult to both understand and to name when incident investigators inevitably encounter them.

How, then, should we seek to structure services that can learn well from incidents?

At the heart of this is an appreciation for the fact that organisations, teams, and systems of work have an unconscious life. It is, perhaps, a transformative intervention to simply accept this as a reality and to reflect upon what it means. Before anything else, therefore, the overarching recommendation from this chapter is that teams and organisations welcome this type of thinking and embrace the relevant literature. Of central importance is the work of Menzies (1961) and her characterisation of unconscious operating principles as 'social defences' which work protectively to try to manage inevitable anxiety. Tom Main (1990) also gives a useful example from the Cassel Hospital of reflection on learning and on noticing the influences that prevent a team from learning well. In this paper, he introduces us to the humility required by leaders to accept that practice is influenced by unconscious processes, meaning, therefore, that they themselves are both vulnerable to these influences and likely to have power involved in the creation and maintenance of them. It is, therefore, a requirement that those who are senior within teams have the emotional resilience to accept the reality of an unconscious life and to involve themselves in its examination.

What helps to nurture this emotional resilience and humility is the acceptance (that comes with an appreciation of an influential unconscious life) of 'the unavoidable reality of anxiety in the workplace' (Barrett, 2020: 128). Barrett (2020) describes the paradigm of 'social defences' (Menzies, 1961) as a 'particularly humane framework for the study of organisations' (128) as it invites an acceptance of the inevitability of powerful emotional influences. Through their study of this field of thought, leaders are, therefore, invited to consider that their skill and effectiveness lies more in curiosity and humility than in infallibility.

The foundational thinking described above provides more than an intellectual space for reflection. It is also about supporting an emotionally containing, psychologically safe culture for staff within which staff experiences are taken seriously and treated as valid. The quality of this 'holding environment' determines the quality of the therapeutic relationship that staff can go onto have with those using the service. It also necessitates an important prerequisite for healthy learning: the provision of protected spaces for reflection within which those uncomfortable aspects of the work which we are powerfully invited to ignore or maintain can be talked and thought about.

**Recommendations for practice**

With this foundation in place, the recommendations from this chapter fall into three broad categories of guided reflection:

1. That when an incident occurs, there is reflection on what was felt by workers to be the primary task at the time. We have outlined in this chapter the importance of task definition and also of how boundaries (such as a clearly defined task) that manage work towards an intended output become easily distorted. Task definition is not, therefore, something which can be achieved and then left. A reflective team which accepts the reality of its own unconscious life should be regularly considering what task their operations and practice serve. This is not to suggest that teams should collapse into accepting the erosion of a stated primary task (shared purpose is an important component of healthy team functioning) but that examination of when and how practice deviated from serving that purpose – with an acceptance that there will be valid, unconscious reasons – is important.
2. That when an incident occurs, there is reflection on what unconscious or invisible principles (or social defences) were in operation at the time. Generally speaking, operating principles should be as transparent as possible for healthy team functioning. Explicit processes allow a team to define its boundaries and act as a buffer against the unconscious social defences which distort them. Deviation from these principles provide teams with a good opportunity to notice something interesting, and healthy teams should be curious about the reasons.
3. That when an incident occurs, the above reflection occurs with a focus on another important boundary – role definition. As before, a curious appreciation for why a role has become unclear or blurred or concerned with tasks which are not those stated in the role description is required.

The importance of the containing culture that surrounds and supports these reflections cannot be overstated. The risk of not providing a safe enough culture which allows for proper reflection is that poor practice is sanctioned.

This section may be well summarised by a quote from Barrett (2020) which seeks to define the characteristics of individuals who form healthy, well-functioning teams:

> They already know what makes for healthy organisational functioning … they get it wrong, things go wrong, they consider their part in it, they learn. They know they are fallible; their knowledge of their fallibility is their strength.
>
> (Barrett, 2020: 132)

**Conclusion**

This chapter is concerned with the inevitability that things will go wrong during our practice as workers within services that care for and manage other human beings. In this regard, this chapter views incidents not as something that can be wholly eradicated through rigorous systemic improvements but as 'red flags' which indicate that compassion and 'patient-centred', humane care has been deviated from. Within a framework that understands organisations as having an unconscious life, these deviations are viewed as also inevitable because of the powerful influences of emotion. It has been argued, therefore, that incidents can be best managed, avoided, and learned from when attention is paid to the needs of workers and teams and to the boundaries which hold the system around them. Humility in leadership is a necessary prerequisite for this type of boundary management which accepts the fallibility of human systems.

## References

Archer, S., Thibaut, B., Dewa, L H., Ramtale, C., D'Lima, D., Simpson, A., Murray, K., Adam, S., & Darzi, A. (2020). Barriers and facilitators to incident reporting in mental healthcare settings: A qualitative study. *Journal of Psychiatric and Mental Health Nursing*, 27(3), 211–223.

Barrett, J. (2020). The Organisation and its Discontents: In search of the fallible and 'good enough' care enterprise. In J. Ramsden, S. Prince, & J. Blazdell (eds), *Working Effectively with 'Personality Disorder': Contemporary and Critical Approaches to Clinical and Organisational Practice.* Shoreham by Sea: Pavilion.

BBC. (2022). 'Toxic culture' of abuse at mental health hospital revealed by BBC secret filming. Panorama team, 28 September. Available from: www.bbc.co.uk/news/uk-63045298

Dixon Woods, M., Baker, R., Charles, K., Dawson, J., Jerzembek, G., Martin, G., McCarthy, I., McKee, L., Minion, L., Ozieranski, P., Willars, J., Wilkie, P., &West, M. (2014). Culture and behaviour in the English National Health Service: Overview of lessons from a large multimethod study. *BMJ Quality and Safety*, 23(2), 106–115.

Heffernan, M. (2013). *Wilful Blindness*. Simon & Schuster.

Hinshelwood, R.D. (2002). Abusive health – helping abuse. The psychodynamic impact of severe personality disorder on caring institutions. *Criminal Behaviour and Mental Health*, 12(S2), S20–S30.

Krantz, S. (1994). Foreword. In A.Obholzer & V. Zagier Roberts, *The Unconscious at Work. Individual and Organizational Stress in the Human Services.* London and New York: Routledge.

Lewis, P.J., & Tully, M.P. (2009). Uncomfortable prescribing conditions in hospitals: The impact of teamwork. *Journal of the Royal Society of Medicine*, 102(11), 481–488.

Lyubovnikova, J., & West, M. (2013). Why teamwork matters: Enabling health care team effectiveness for the delivery of high-quality patient care. In E. Salas, S. Tannenbaum, D. Cohen, & G. Latham (eds), *Developing and Enhancing Teamwork in Organizations* (pp.331–372). San Francisco, CA: Jossey-Bass.

Lyubovnikova, J., West, M. A., Dawson, J.F., & Carter, M.R. (2015). 24-Karat or fools gold? Consequences of real team and co-acting group membership in healthcare organisations. *European Journal of Work and Organizational Psychology*, 24(6), 929–950.

Main, T. (1990). Knowledge, learning and freedom from thought. *Psychoanalytic Psychotherapy*, 5(1), 59–74.

Menzies, I. (1961). The functioning of social systems as a defense against anxiety. Human *Relations*, 13, 95–121.

Miller, E. J., & Rice, A. K. (1967). *Systems of Organisation.* London: Tavistock.

Mid Staffordshire NHS Foundation Trust Public Inquiry. (2013). *Report of the Mid Staffordshire NHS Foundation Trust Public Inquiry: Executive summary.* Available from: www.gov.uk/government/publications/report-of-the-mid-staffordshire-nhs-foundation-trust-public-inquiry

Nembhard, I. M., & Edmondson, A. C. (2006). Making it safe. The effects of leader inclusiveness and professional status on psychological safety and improvement efforts in healthcare teams. *Journal of Organisational Behaviour*, 27(7), 941–966.

NHS England. (2022). The national speak up policy. Available from: www.england.nhs.uk/publication/the-national-speak-up-policy

Obholzer, A., & Zagier Roberts, V. (eds) (1994). *The Unconscious at Work: Individual and Organizational Stress in the Human Services.* London and New York: Routledge.

Ross, F., Rink, E., & Fern, A. (2000). Integration or pragmatic coalition? An evaluation of nursing teams in primary care. *Journal of Interprofessional Care*, 14(3), 259–267.

Stokes, J. (1994). The unconscious at work in groups and teams. Contributions from the work of Wilfred Bion. In A. Obholzer & V. Zagier Roberts (eds), *The Unconscious at Work: Individual and Organizational Stress in the Human Services.* London and New York: Routledge.

Zagier Roberts, V. (1994). The organisation of work: Contributions from open systems theory. In A. Obholzer & V. Zagier Roberts (eds), *The Unconscious at Work: Individual and Organizational Stress in the Human Services.* London & New York: Routledge.

**PART 4**

# Post-investigation reporting, learning, and development

## 15 Approaches to managing information post investigation

*Jenny Shaw*

### Introduction

This chapter discusses the preparing, processing, and prioritising of investigative data, as the generation of this information will fundamentally influence the direction and outcome of the investigation (Vrij et al., 2014). Its aim is to assist investigators in identifying what information is required to complete the investigation. It will examine the types of information available and enable an appreciation of how this can help frame the investigation in question. This includes the practicalities of access and the importance of proportionality when using this information during the investigation. It will move on to the aspects to consider when 'fact finding', what types of information may be included, and the importance of critical and systematic analysis. The chapter concludes with an examination of contextual factors to consider when managing information.

What do we mean by information? Information is defined by the Oxford English Dictionary (2023) as 'Knowledge communicated concerning some particular fact, subject, or event; that of which one is apprised or told'. In terms of serious incident investigation, this could be the facts surrounding an individual, situation, event/s, organisations, and associated circumstances. However, this statement does not illustrate or highlight the complexities of dealing with, managing, and interpreting facts generally and specifically in an incident investigation. The chapter will examine this area and the issues of objectivity and subjectivity, including their relevance in the investigation process.

To understand how we manage information in investigations, we need a conceptual framework, such as root cause analysis (Balakrishnan et al., 2019), a human factors, or a systems-based approach (Weaver et al., 2021), such as the Systems Engineering Initiative for Patient Safety (SEIPS) approach (Holden et al., 2013) which is endorsed by the Patient Safety Incident Response Framework (NHS England, 2022a). The framework of investigations, the purpose and remit of the investigation, influences the information required, so we cannot isolate information from the purpose of its acquisition.

DOI: 10.4324/9781003286240-20

## Developing an awareness of the evidence required

At the start of any investigation, the terms of reference indicate the scope and the boundaries of the examination and analysis of the incident or event. The importance of scope and terms of reference cannot be overestimated (Väth et al., 2023), as they provide a fundamental framework and authority for the investigators. 'Typical' terms of reference, whether in health, social care, or other areas of practice, should be able to qualify the following to support the investigation process (Kelsey, 2023). These include and are not limited to the following

- **The time period to be investigated.** This includes its scope, be it over a period of months or years, depending on the nature of the event under investigation.
- **The areas and matters under review and examination.** These can include the quality of care and treatment of the individual/s at the centre of the investigation, staff supervision, training and skills, system organisation and processes both internally and externally, and compliance with the organisation's policies and procedures, relevant guidelines, and regulations. It also may include environmental factors which may have impacted on the event or incident. This last area is in line with the human factors approach to investigations (Broadribb, 2012) as discussed in a Chapter 3.
- **The ultimate outcome of the investigation including the completion of a report, recommendations and lessons learned.** Investigators need to be mindful of the internal and external policies and forums and the wider audience for their final report.
- **The period for completion of the investigation.** This is dependent on current internal and external guidelines and practices.

It should be remembered that terms of reference can be dependent on specific requirements requested following the instigation of the investigative process (Kelsey, 2023). However, the above overview of the format of investigations illustrates the key and constant areas to be included in all processes.

## Access to materials and people – practicalities

Once the scope, purpose, and process of the investigation are outlined and agreed, the next step is to plan how to obtain access to the information and to the relevant people/professionals as part of the initial stages of the process. We will move on to types of information which would be useful later in the chapter. However, a prior stage is to consider how to gain access to any relevant information. The practical questions to ask at the start of an investigation, based on the author's experience of undertaking investigations, include:

- How can the information be obtained? What processes are in place to support the request? Is there a time constraint in obtaining information which may impact on the completion of the investigation report?

- Is information required from outside the organisation? If so, what type of information? Is it central to, and identified in, the scope of the investigation? How will it aid and support the analysis of information and investigators in identifying key areas and themes? Is there a data-sharing agreement in place between organisations which can facilitate information between organisations? Is there a multi-agency approach to investigations which involve each party? Are there any barriers to obtaining records, documentation, and access to staff? If so, how can these be resolved?

What other methods of obtaining information need to be considered? Are interviews required? If so, why, and what can only be obtained via this methodology, or is there an alternative way of obtaining this information (Driskell & Salas, 2015)? What is the organisational process for staff interviews, and how will staff be supported, as involvement in adverse events can have a traumatic impact on those involved (Seys et al., 2013)? Interviews may be overwhelming for some individuals and can prove counterproductive in obtaining the necessary information (Madsen & Holmberg, 2015). It is important to remember the distinction between specialised interviews as part of an investigative and informative approach after an incident and those that are part of a formal procedure, such as a human resources issue. The purpose and scope of the interview, including the areas requiring discussion, need to be specific and within the interviewee's practice remit and knowledge expertise to respond:

- As acknowledged in previous chapters, the involvement of the individual central to the investigation (where appropriate and depending on the circumstances of the incident) is important and essential. It helps to understand their perspective and experiences of their involvement and, significantly, their view of the incident. By including this information, the subsequent findings and report have enhanced validity and relevance. However, in specific investigations, such as with homicide reviews, it may not be possible to contact or interview the person, for many reasons, including the current stage of any criminal justice procedure, specifically if a homicide incident, and the wider implications of the event being investigated. We need to acknowledge how we have aimed to include those directly involved and how we have attempted to include their views and personal account in the final report.
- In addition to the information which can be obtained by the person/s central to the event/incident, the data collected from the family and significant parties can be invaluable. What information would be useful and needed? This question is about any background personal and social information, their experiences of services and/or organisations, and their views on how systems and issues can be improved and resolved. Reference has already been made to the duty of candour requirement in this book, but it would be additionally beneficial for investigators to ensure inclusion of families, carers, and significant others in the recommendations or improvement actions identified. The Patient Safety Incident Response Framework (PSIRF) (NHS England, 2022b) has, as a key driving

principle and standard, the involvement and engagement of those involved in any incident, be it the person receiving the care or treatment, their family or carers, and the staff members.

- Given the move to a new framework, specifically in the NHS and the new PSIRF, with reference to a wider human factors and systems approaches, are there opportunities to instigate a new more collaborative methodology, such as peer discussion and focus group? Would this be in line with an approach which is system-wide and encompasses lessons learned, a practical system theory approach to incidents and adverse events?

The above questions and points serve as a checklist to consider at the start of the process and are to be viewed as a reflective aid. However, the emphasis is now on a wider collaborative perspective and examination, so it is advantageous to consider various information methodologies.

A constant theme is the reason for the investigation. The approach to be adopted is dependent on its remit, the scope, the areas of investigation, and the roles of those charged with leading the inquiry. It is also reliant on the individual factors pertinent to the event. These considerations lead into the next section of the chapter.

### Understanding the organisational culture, its role, and impact on information management

All organisations, their purpose, structure, and function have an influence on the investigation process (Hopkins, 2006), This is both explicit and implicit. Whilst the organisational culture and ethos should not directly impact on why and how investigations are conducted, it is a reality that this can be a component in the management and process of investigations. How this translates into the practice of incident investigation varies between and across organisations.

What do we mean by organisational cultural information context? The cultural backdrop of organisations (whether NHS, social care, independent, third sector, or criminal justice) relates not only to the governance surrounding the obtaining of information and the approval of the final investigation report, but significantly to how they ensure that any lessons learned and recommendations made are considered and adopted (Ullström et al., 2014). Whilst this is not within the scope of this chapter, it is essential when considering specifically how the organisation will mobilise and complete the implementation of recommendations.

When examining a cross-system investigation, it is important to appreciate and place in context the role of each agency and how their available information can inform the incident information gathering and analysis.

### The importance of event chronology and timelines – how they help understanding the information and how we use information to guide the investigation

We have considered in this chapter the wider-ranging and generic areas of the information process. There is one significant aspect of information management that is crucial to how the investigation progresses, the identification of findings and themes, any responsibility which requires additional oversight, and ultimately the lessons identified and the recommendations made. Without a clear overview and understanding of what happened and when, a thorough and objective overview of the incident would be difficult to acquire or make sense of. By completing a comprehensive timeline, we can understand what occurred and why, areas of good and poor practice, what are the gaps in information, an overview of themes and significant issues (Momen et al., 2013). The importance of the chronology cannot not be dismissed. It is an area which investigators need to spend a considerable time in collating and interpreting. It forms the backbone of the report.

What do we mean when referring to a chronology or timeline? How far should our reference to the fundamental episodes in an involvement with services or systems extend? What it is not, or shouldn't be, is a reproduction or copy of existing records and/ or clinical notes. A chronology and timeline should provide a narrative and picture of each significant contact, session, communication, and event leading up to the incident or event. To achieve this, as investigators, we need to understand the complexity of each incidence and time period within the context of the practitioner, their organisational policies, the practice framework in place, any agencies involved and inter-agency working, and the contact with the people central to the event (Shortland et al., 2020).

Below are some key factors to remember when completing the chronology, what to include, what to summarise, and what to append.

Central to this process is an understanding of *fact management*. By this, we mean the ability to understand a variety of sources of information and data, and place them in the context of the event to 'tell the narrative'. This should also identify the themes and core learning, and enable practitioners and organisations to act upon the improvement recommendations highlighted.

The narrative should provide a description and analysis of the individual's journey through services. This includes what worked well and above recognised best practice and evidence-based practice, areas which demonstrated good communication and collaboration between the person, their family/carers, and professionals involved in the delivery of care and treatment.

The timeline has a function in providing the factual basis for further analysis and clarification, identifying specific areas where additional information and inquiry is required (Hope et al., 2013).

At the start, this process can be divided into key stages; the 'what?', how we summarise areas within the report, and what can be included as appendices.

## The 'what?'

Reference has been made to the types and various approaches to obtaining information This includes the use of group forums, multi-disciplinary team discussion and analysis, and supportive investigation techniques such as After-Action Reviews (AARs) (Villado & Arthur, 2013). The list of potential documentation and records to be examined may be vast. The initial stages of information management will consider the circumstances of the incident and can help determine a view of the material to be accessed. This includes clinical/care records as previously mentioned, in addition to the policies and procedures that were in place at the time of the incident or event. It is additionally helpful to consider the usefulness of report templates and frameworks for the report in guiding the management of the material and information.

## Summaries

An important area is how we summarise key information in the final report and the rationale for its inclusion. This often incorporates the background history of the patient/person who uses services, so consideration should be given to how their information should be presented, ideally with the involvement of their family/carers. When completing the report and from the information examined, it is important to consider the development of the narrative and why a particular aspect needs to be included. Does it help provide context to the event? Does it form a key explanation of events, which then leads to the identification of an area of improvement arising from the incident? We often examine extensive records and clinical information concerning an individual or a service and may be 'tempted' to reiterate that level of detail in the report. However, it is useful to reflect on whether such detail aids in understanding the circumstances and supports the investigation's findings and conclusions. This is a beneficial technique to adopt in other sections of the report to ensure that it meets the aims as outlined in the terms of reference.

## Appendices

Why do we need appendices and what purpose do they serve? These relate to those documents that can aid and support the narrative and findings of the report. This can include the methodology and approaches adopted in examining and analysing the information gathered. Examples include fishbone diagrams and explanatory guides and references which have been documented in the main report.

## When to stop

During any investigation, it is not uncommon to be surrounded by documents, statements from interviews, policies, national and local guidance, clinical documentation, records such as letters, emails, training records, and so on. We feel the need to have all this information to find out what happened and why. However, we need to be realistic and question how much information is needed to meet the scope and purpose of the investigation. The wider considerations when examining various sources of information include the following examples and areas to reflect on during the investigation:

### *Systematic review and critique of material*

- Terms of reference revisited – to ensure that we have addressed all areas as outlined.

- Causation v lessons learned – recognising the new approach in the PSIRF (NHS England, 2022b).
- Hindsight bias (Groß & Bayen, 2022) – recognising that we are examining information after the event.
- Subjectivity and objectivity – the balance to be achieved in information analysis.
- Themes and how they inform recommendations and actions – this includes reference to any wider organisational thematic analysis (Braun & Clarke, 2012) and an examination of similar incidents and events to highlight trends and themes.

### *Contextual factors*

- Organisational factors and dynamics to be considered as part of the situational background.
- The wider demographics and socio-economic context.

## Conclusion

This chapter has provided an overview of the information available and required during incident investigations. It also acknowledges the need to consider the specific circumstances surrounding events, their context, the acquisition of the views and perspective of those directly involved, and the organisational practice and ethos. This is whilst being mindful of the scope of the investigation itself.

## References

Balakrishnan, K., Brenner, M. J., Gosbee, J. W., & Schmalbach, C. E. (2019). Patient Safety/ Quality Improvement Primer, Part II: Prevention of Harm Through Root Cause Analysis and Action (RCA2). *Otolaryngology – Head and Neck Surgery*, 161(6), 911–921.

Braun, V., & Clarke, V. (2012). Thematic analysis. In H. Cooper (ed.) *APA Handbook of Research Methods in Psychology, Vol. 2, Research Designs*, pp. 57–71. Washington, DC: APA Books.

Broadribb, M. P. (2012). It's people, stupid! Human factors in incident investigation. *Process Safety Progress*, 31(2), 152–158.

Driskell, T., & Salas, E. (2015). Investigative Interviewing: Harnessing the Power of the Team. *Group Dynamics*, 19(4), 273–289.

Groß, J., & Bayen, U. J. (2022). Older and younger adults' hindsight bias after positive and negative outcomes. *Memory & Cognition*, 50(1), 16–28.

Holden, R. J., Carayon, P., Gurses, A. P., Hoonakker, P., Hundt, A. S., Ozok, A. A., & Rivera-Rodriguez, A. J. (2013). SEIPS 2.0: A human factors framework for studying and improving the work of healthcare professionals and patients. *Ergonomics*, 56 (11), 1669–1686.

Hope, L., Mullis, R., & Gabbert, F. (2013). Who? What? When? Using a timeline technique to facilitate recall of a complex event. *Journal of Applied Research in Memory and Cognition*, 2(1), 20–24.

Hopkins, A. (2006). Studying organisational cultures and their effects on safety. *Safety Science*, 44(10), 875–889.

Kelsey, R. (2023). *Patient Safety: Investigating and Reporting Serious Clinical Incidents* (2nd ed.). CRC Press.

Madsen, K., & Holmberg, U. (2015). Interviewees' Psychological Well-being in Investigative Interviews: A Therapeutic Jurisprudential Approach. *Psychiatry, Psychology, and Law*, 22(1), 60–74.

Momen, N., Kendall, M., Barclay, S., & Murray, S. (2013). Using timelines to depict patient journeys: A development for research methods and clinical care review. *Primary Health Care Research & Development*, 14(4), 403–408.

NHS England (2022a). *Patient Safety Incident Response Framework; Supporting Guidance, Guide to responding proportionately to patient safety incidents,* NHS England, Version 1.

NHS England (2022b). *Patient Safety Incident Response Framework Supporting Guidance, Engaging and involving patients, families and staff following a patient safety incident.* NHS England, Learning Together, and Healthcare Safety Investigation Branch, Version 1.

Oxford English Dictionary. (2023) Reference. Available from: www.oed.com/view/Entry/160845

Seys, D., Scott, S., Wu, A., Van Gerven, E., Vleugels, A., Euwema, M., Panella, M., Conway, J., Sermeus, W., & Vanhaecht, K. (2013). Supporting involved health care professionals (second victims) following an adverse health event: A literature review. *International Journal of Nursing Studies*, 50(5), 678–687.

Shortland, N., Alison, L., Thompson, L., Barrett-Pink, C., & Swan, L. (2020). Choice and consequence: A naturalistic analysis of least-worst decision-making in critical incidents. *Memory & Cognition*, 48(8), 1334–1345.

Ullström, S., Andreen Sachs, M., Hansson, J., Øvretveit, J., & Brommels, M. (2014). Suffering in silence: A qualitative study of second victims of adverse events. *BMJ Quality & Safety*, 23(4), 325–331.

Väth, S. J., Flaig, M., & Gaus, H. (2023). Terms of reference matter – insights from evaluations of Finnish development cooperation. *Zeitschrift Für Evaluation*, 22(1), 39–54.

Villado, A. J., & Arthur, W. (2013). The Comparative Effect of Subjective and Objective After-Action Reviews on Team Performance on a Complex Task. *Journal of Applied Psychology*, 98(3), 514–528.

Vrij, A., Hope, L., & Fisher, R. P. (2014). Eliciting Reliable Information in Investigative Interviews. *Policy Insights from the Behavioral and Brain Sciences,* 1(1), 129–136.

Weaver, S., Stewart, K., & Kay, L. (2021). Systems-based investigation of patient safety incidents. *Future Healthcare Journal*, 8(3), e593–e597.

# 16 How to present a report and the executive summary

*Teresa Lean*

This chapter will focus on the sharing and dissemination of investigation reports within the service affected and the tools to support and share information with a focus on the National Health Service (NHS) although the investigative process and the principles are largely transferable to other agencies and institutions. The development of two documents is crucial to the reporting of the investigation outcomes: a detailed report and an executive summary, which is brief and accessible. There are several key documents that underpin the approach and provide a guide to both the investigation and the report. These will be referenced throughout and include NHS England's Serious Incident Framework Policy (2010, revised 2015) which defines incidents requiring investigation as 'events in health care where the potential for learning is so great, or the consequences to patients, families and carers, staff or organisations are so significant, that they warrant using additional resources to mount a comprehensive response' (NHS England, 2015: 12). With over 1.4 million patient safety incidents reported annually (Peerally et al., 2022), it is crucial that those meeting the criteria for investigation are recorded across organisations using the systems and services commissioned by NHS England, typically the Serious Incidents Requiring Investigation Framework (SIRI). However, this framework has been replaced by the Patient Safety Incident Response Framework (PSIRF) (NHS England, 2022) which was introduced in August 2022, and the chapter will conclude with an overview of that framework.

When incidents occur, it is imperative that we adopt a process that robustly identifies the background and context of the incident to analyse the care and treatment provided and identify factors that contributed to or influenced the outcome (NHS England, 2015). Organisations must learn from serious incidents to reduce the risk of the same incident occurring again. However, there are often recurring themes amongst reported incidents which would suggest that learning does not always occur; this risks overwhelming the organisation to such a degree that it makes the thorough investigation of incidents unachievable (Archer et al., 2017). Investigations require a considerable amount of both time and resources, so the organisation needs to ensure that there is an appropriate balance between the resources being used to investigate and report on the incident and the resources needed to implement and embed learning to reduce the likelihood of the incident happening again (NHS England, 2015).

DOI: 10.4324/9781003286240-21

Patient care and treatment is the ultimate priority of the NHS and health and social care providers. Any incident that causes harm must be investigated to ensure that any further risk is mitigated (NHS England, 2019). Patients must always be fully informed of the outcome of the investigation. Any incident that results in death or serious harm should include family and carers in the investigation (NHS England, 2020) to give them opportunity to express their concerns about what went wrong and to give feedback on outcomes. An investigation is not and should never be an interrogation; it is therefore imperative that families are treated with compassion and dignity with an open, honest, and transparent approach from the organisation itself (see Chapter 4). The investigation lead should remain objective, report fairly and without prejudice, and always act in patients' best interests and safeguard where necessary (Grimes, 2021).

When writing the investigation report, it is first necessary to give a brief description of the component parts of the report. These may vary between organisations; however, the basic structure should remain the same. Although the executive summary sits at the front of the report, it is written last, as it is a summary of what follows. This chapter will move on to focus on the importance of the executive summary itself and what it should contain and why.

To provide a focus to the writing of a serious incident investigation report, the following hypothetical scenario will be referred to throughout the chapter:

A patient with a diagnosis of psychosis was admitted to the ward after experiencing auditory hallucinations and paranoid beliefs. The patient quickly deteriorated on the ward. Due to sickness and the use of agency staff, they did not know the patient well and were unfamiliar with his presentation and symptoms. The patient allegedly assaulted a member of staff after believing they wanted to cause him harm.

### Incident on a page

This is exactly as its name suggests. Such a brief incident report should clearly identify the type of incident that has met the 'serious investigation' criteria (e.g. disruptive/aggressive/violent behaviour). It should identify the specific group of staff it relates to (e.g. inpatient staff), and it should concisely identify what happened, any areas of good practice, the learning points, and what that staff group needs to do in future. So, if the incident occurred because the patient was extremely unwell and had displayed aggressive behaviour in response to auditory hallucinations, it may include urgent risk assessment of the patient's presenting condition and request for an earlier medic review. It should also identify links to resources or references for similar incidents.

### Duty of candour

Organisations should always show their commitment to being open and honest. Duty of candour is a statutory requirement which includes telling the relevant person as soon as practically possible once a patient safety incident has occurred (NHS England, 2015). Offering an apology has historically been viewed as an acceptance of guilt;

however, this is not the case. An apology should be offered promptly and in a meaningful way which fully explains what has happened when an incident has occurred.

This section of the report also details the name of the allocated investigation lead whose responsibility it is to keep the patient and their family members up to date with the progress of the investigation. They are also a point of contact for the family to raise concerns; any concerns they do raise must be included within the body of the actual report.

It is not always possible to complete duty of candour, especially if the patient is very unwell, does not have any family, or has been excommunicated by their family. In such cases, safeguarding advice should always be sought.

## Terms of reference

These are agreed by the lead investigating manager in conjunction with the investigation team. Every incident report should include the following general terms of reference, establishing the facts of what happened, to whom, when, where, how, and why. Establish if there were any other agencies involved in the care and treatment of the patient, and how and why they were involved. All parties involved in the provision of care and treatment should be included in the learning review. A commitment to identifying omissions in the provision of care and treatment must be present, with further commitment to establishing any root causes or contributing factors. Furthermore, the terms of reference should ensure that the investigation aims to identify that care and treatment complied with statutory obligations, best practice guidance, and local operational policies.

Terms of reference must also include identifying lessons for learning, and what the recommendations are for the action plan to improve systems and services to reduce the risk of future harm to other patients. It should also commit to sharing the outcome of the investigation with all relevant parties. If we use the example above of disruptive/aggressive/violent behaviour, additional and specific terms of reference would include questions such as 'Did adequate escalation take place on signs of relapse?', 'Did the presence of auditory hallucinations increase risk to others?', and 'Was a review of as required (PRN) medication indicated?'

## Scope of investigation

This should provide a simple factual statement to say that the investigation examined the care and treatment of the patient between the specific dates, usually the date of admission to the date of the incident. The report then needs to further state that it has examined the events that took place in detail, including contributory factors. At this point, it commits to providing recommendations to address the issues identified.

## Information and evidence gathered

This section identifies the resources used by the investigation lead, which will include the reporting system and the clinical note recording systems. It should document the name of any policies or guidelines that have been used to measure best practice against, such as service operation procedures (SOPs). It should also include an anonymised list of people involved in the incident, including their role and whether each of those people have provided a statement. Closed-circuit television, if available, should also be referenced.

## Investigation methodology

This details the framework that has been used to analyse the incident such as the Yorkshire contributory factors framework, which was developed by human factor experts. Its use supports the identification of contributory factors in patient safety incidents to optimise learning and reduce future risk. It aims to improve patient safety by looking at how systems work and how the complexity of both environmental and individual factors impact on patient safety (Heier et al., 2021).

## Background and context

This should include basic patient information and demographics, including personal social history, medication, past medical history, and any recent routine bloods and investigations. It should also include a concise psychiatric history and concordance with prescribed medication. The investigating officer should be looking to identify times or areas of care and treatment where there was enough concern to have taken action to minimise the risk of any harm to self or others occurring.

## Chronology of care and treatment

This is a concise timeline of events detailing what happened and when. It should identify the source of the information and any concerns found. This begins to build a picture of how the investigation will be carried out, who needs to be spoken to, any policies or guidance that need to be referred to. It includes the point at which risks could/should have been identified and whether appropriate action was taken to mitigate the risk – in other words, what was the probability of an unwanted event (Nathan et al., 2021)?

## Service/care delivery problems and contributory factors

This section then looks at the summary of the findings using the contributory factors framework. Using the aforementioned domains, it looks specifically at situation factors including team factors (was there appropriate leadership at the time?), individual staff factors (were staff up to date with training?), task characteristics (failure to recognise a deteriorating patient), and patient factors (symptoms of psychosis).

Local working conditions should be taken into consideration including workload and staffing issues (reduced staffing levels/use of agency staff), together with leadership, supervision, and staff roles (poor coordination of a response to a patient's deteriorating health), and drugs, equipment, and supplies (was a medical review or medication review requested?).

Organisation factors would include the physical environment itself (was it appropriate for a deteriorating patient?), support from other departments (was there any?), scheduling and bed management (was a bed available if admission/transfer indicated?), and staff training and education (was it up to date?).

External factors need to be considered, such as the design of equipment, supplies and drugs (was as-needed medication utilised effectively?). A record of which national policies were adhered to requires mentioning if indicated.

The final domain looks at culture and communication: safety culture (recognition of how to keep patients safe) and verbal and written communication (could this be improved to highlight risk, recognise symptoms, and therefore reduce risk?).

### Analysis of care and treatment including contributing or influencing factors identified

This should all be comprehensively and concisely written in the above at this point of the report, without further need to elaborate.

### Response to questions raised by the patient/family

The NHS national constitution for England 2015 (NHS England, 2023) states that patients will be at the heart of everything that the NHS does and that it is accountable to the public, communities, and patients that is serves. It also states that the NHS will actively encourage feedback from the public, patients, and staff, welcome it, and use it to improve its services.

Involving the family is not only ethically and morally justified but also necessary for acceptance. It can support the grieving process and re-establish bonds of trust, especially if the patient or family has a different perspective from the professional perspective. The family can offer insights that may have been overlooked, adding valuable knowledge that can inform learning from what has gone wrong (Kok et al., 2018).

Have the family's concerns been adequately addressed and were they shared by others? For example, a concern may have been raised around timely and adequate intervention for a deteriorating patient, which might have reduced or mitigated the harm caused. Is the patient or family in agreement with the findings?

### Root cause(s)

What are the root causes? The process of root cause analysis is used to reduce patient safety incidents, which can be achieved when the factors influencing the incident are identified and addressed (Alifa & Dhamanti, 2022). It may be that earlier intervention would have mitigated or reduced risk, and that a failure to recognise a deteriorating patient and request a medic review resulted in the incident, which might have been avoidable.

## Conclusion

This report conclusion should both summarise and acknowledge historical risks based on previous psychiatric history including possible risks of disengagement, poor medication concordance, increased symptoms, and lack of review, all of which may contribute to increased risk.

## Lessons learned and sharing learning from the investigation

This should already be detailed in the 'Incident on a page' section. But it should detail here how that information will be disseminated and in what format.

## Recommendations

List the recommendations in priority order, despite many recommendations having equal priority. Examples include reviewing escalation plans for when a patient deteriorates and training for staff around as-needed medication.

## Support provided to staff involved

This is a key area of any investigation and often a contentious issue in relation to perceived support versus actual support. It is often quoted that asking staff to provide statements immediately after an incident can cause re-traumatisation. However, failure to do so risks poor memory recall and/or a collective recollection of the incident once the team members have discussed it amongst themselves (Braun et al., 2021). That is not to say that there is a deliberate intention to collude to distort the facts, but it risks distortion or failure to report the incident factually. Furthermore, support for staff is crucial in terms of recruitment and retention, future risk management, and commitment to the organisation (Sato & Kodama, 2021).

## Action plan

The action plan should list all the recommendations and the specific actions to be completed. It should identify the measure to be used and what the impact of that will be, how it will be achieved, what relevance it has in terms of improving practice and reducing risk, when it will be achieved, who the action owner is, and whether the action is classed as strong, intermediate, or weak. An example for a recommendation of training for staff on the use of as-needed medication would include pharmacy staff to deliver an education session to staff on planning the use of PRN medications at multidisciplinary meetings and how to recognise, record, and communicate symptoms. This would increase effective management of symptoms and can be audited. It would occur at the multidisciplinary team level and provide opportunity to support a deteriorating patient in a timelier manner to reduce the distress of symptoms and risk to self or others. The action owner may be the senior nursing manager and classed as intermediate.

**Glossary**

Depending upon the use of legal, technical, or clinical language, a glossary may be needed to enhance accessibility and comprehension.

**Revision history**

This is another important aspect of the report as it details the history of report versions, when it has been revised, and any changes made and by whom. Apart from the investigation lead, this could include the patient safety team and clinical governance lead. It is crucial that updated versions of the report are circulated by one person as often several versions can be in circulation, which causes great confusion particularly for the investigation lead when they are questioned on an earlier report action that has subsequently been updated.

This section concludes the main report.

**Executive summary**

Once the main report has been written, the investigation lead can then write the executive summary. This is in essence the most important part of the investigation report and needs to be accessible and concise. It should provide a concise chronology of the care and treatment, detail the facts leading up to the incident and who was involved, and identify any lessons learned to help prevent further incidents of the same nature. It should also aim to improve the reporting and investigation of future serious events. The executive summary always sits at the front of the report and is the first section to be read at the safety summit, which is a meeting of key stakeholders in the organisation who come together to discuss and review the information within the report, and who agree the actions needed because of the risks identified (NHS England, 2017). This will also be read by the coroner and, most importantly, the patient and family. It should not include any information that is not in the body of the report, and it should give the reader a clear indication of what happened.

As stated at the beginning of the chapter, it is necessary to point out that the Serious Incident Framework (NHS England, 2015) has been replaced by the Patient Safety Incident Response Framework (2022) which does not distinguish between 'patient safety incidents' and 'serious incidents'. Instead, it advocates for the allocation of resources to be balanced with the resources needed to deliver improvements to reduce risk, offering a more proportionate approach. It is less of a prescriptive investigation framework and more of a responsive approach that advocates engaging with those affected by incidents in a more compassionate way, to embed a culture of patient safety in a system of improvement (NHS England, 2022). This approach should align with the NHS Constitution and its vision for healthcare services to actively welcome and encourage feedback from the public, patients, and staff and use it to improve its service (NHS England, 2023).

## References

Alifia, R. T., & Dhamanti, I. (2022). Implementation of root cause analysis on patient safety incidence in hospital: Literature review. *Journal of Public Health Research and Community Health Development*, 6(1), 14–20.

Archer, S., Hull, L., Soukup, T., Mayer, E., Athanasiou, T., Sevdalis, N., & Darzi, A. (2017). Development of a theoretical framework of factors affecting patient safety incident reporting: A theoretical review of the literature. *British Medical Journal Open*, 7(12), e017155.

Braun, B. E., Zaragoza, M. S., Chrobak, Q. M., & Ithisuphalap, J. (2021). Correcting eyewitness suggestibility: Does explanatory role predict resistance to correction? *Memory*, 29(1), 59–77.

Grimes, J. E. (2021). *Investigative Interviewing: Adopting a Forensic Mindset.* CRC Press.

Heier, L., Riouchi, D., Hammerschmidt, J., Gambashidze, N., Kocks, A., & Ernstmann, N. (2021). Safety performance in acute medical care: A qualitative, explorative study on the perspectives of healthcare professionals. *Healthcare*, 9(11), 1543.

Kok, J., Leistikow, I., & Bal, R. (2018). Patient and family engagement in incident investigations: Exploring hospital manager and incident Investigating Officer experiences and challenges. *Journal of Health Services Research & Policy*, 23(4), 252–261.

Nathan, R., Whyler, J., & Wilson, P. (2021). Risk of harm to others: Subjectivity and meaning of risk in mental health practice. *Journal of Risk Research*, 24(10), 1228–1238.

NHS England. (2015). *Serious Incident Framework: Supporting learning to prevent recurrence.* Available from: www.england.nhs.uk/wp-content/uploads/2015/04/serious-incidnt-framwrk-upd.pdf

NHS England. (2017). *Risks Summits: National Guidance.* Available from: www.england.nhs.uk/wp-content/uploads/2017/07/risk-summit-guidance-july-2017.pdf

NHS England. (2019). *The NHS Patient Safety Strategy.* Available from: www.england.nhs.uk/patient-safety/the-nhs-patient-safety-strategy

NHS England. (2020). *NRLS national patient safety incident reports: commentary.* Available from: www.england.nhs.uk/publication/nrls-national-patient-safety-incident-reports-commentary-september-2020

NHS England. (2022). *Patient safety incident response framework.* Available from: www.england.nhs.uk/publication/patient-safety-incident-response-framework-and-supporting-guidance

NHS England. (2023). *The NHS Constitution for England.* Available from: www.gov.uk/government/publications/the-nhs-constitution-for-england/the-nhs-constitution-for-england

National Patient Safety Agency. (2009). *Being Open: Communicating Patient Safety Incidents with Patients, Their Families and Carers.* London: HMSO.

Peerally, M. F., Carr, S., Waring, J., Martin, G., & Dixon-Woods, M. (2022). A content analysis of contributory factors reported in serious incident investigation reports in hospital care. *Clinical Medicine*, 22(5), 423–433.

Sato, K., & Kodama, Y. (2021). Nurses' educational needs when dealing with aggression from patients and their families: A mixed-methods study. *British Medical Journal*, 11(1), e041711.

# 17 Cautionary tales

## Investigations – the effects on staff involved

*Panchu Xavier*

'No one comes into the caring profession to cause harm … clinicians are only human.' We have heard this said during 'investigations' into serious untoward incidents in the National Health Service (NHS) but still we hear of clinicians being adversely affected by the process of learning from a serious incident review.

All over the world, healthcare providers know that patients who come into healthcare facilities have a chance of coming to harm. It was in the year 2000 that the article 'To err is human' was published following a study in the USA by the Institute of Medicine (Havens & Boroughs, 2000), which showed that over 98,000 individuals died because of medical errors in hospitals yearly. A truly shocking figure when you consider that American healthcare providers are known for world-leading use of technology and safety systems. There are similar reviews from the United Kingdom (Panagioti et al., 2019) that show that there is preventable harm taking place in 1 in 20 healthcare interventions.

The World Health Organization's Safety Update (2019) highlighted the extent of preventable deaths taking place in developed and developing nations. According to this report, there are an estimated 2.6 million deaths in low- and middle-income countries due to medical errors every year. The numbers are simply too large to fathom and accept. But it is something that we must all bear in mind: the impact of poorly designed services and systems that do not allow flawed humans, as we all are, to work safely in them. However, the publication 'An Organisation with a memory' by Donaldson (2002: 3) speaks about the potential impact of having safer systems on patient safety incidents. A key moment in NHS patient safety history.

Unfortunately, we have multiple examples from the United Kingdom of how poor care and poor systems led to serious harm to patients. The Mid Staffordshire Inquiry report by Robert Francis (2013) and the Morecambe Bay Investigation report by Bill Kirkup (2015) are just two examples of inquiries commissioned by health secretaries to investigate poor outcomes in the NHS. These two reports highlighted what happens when there is a lack of clarity around responsibility and accountability in organisations.

The Mid Staffordshire Inquiry reported the appalling stories of patients who had been harmed by poor care because of a 'serious failure on the part of a provider Trust Board' (Francis, 2013: 3). The report noted how the organisation did not listen to patients and staff or act on the concerns that were raised to them.

DOI: 10.4324/9781003286240-22

The harsh criticism of the Trust was summed up by Sir Robert Francis: 'Above all, it failed to tackle an insidious negative culture involving a tolerance of poor standards and a disengagement from managerial and leadership responsibilities' (3). A damming indictment of the numerous systems and processes that were set up to ensure that patient care was the best. This shocking account of poor care took place at the time when multiple organisations, including NHS commissioners, Monitor, professional bodies, who were all tasked with ensuring that standards were maintained and patients were not harmed, failed in their duties. We have spoken about how a culture of an organisation helps its staff be open and honest about concerns in the quality of care delivered. Here was an example of how the culture was one in which the organisation placed the achievement of positive information and financial independence above quality standards and positive outcomes for patients. The report criticises the NHS Trust for its self-promotion, when it should have been reflecting and learning from its mistakes, its poor governance, and professionals being disengaged. The NHS Trust appeared to be to focusing its resources on achieving its foundation trust (FT) status – FTs have more freedom to run their business – and may have lost sight of other priorities at that time.

The recommendations in the Francis Report are far-reaching and have led to significant improvements in the NHS since its publication. The then Health Secretary Jeremy Hunt spoke a year later about the improvements in the NHS that resulted from the Francis Report, referred to as the 'Francis effect' (Department of Health and Social Care, 2014). There was a move away from financial targets to one in which the patient is placed at the centre of care, and Trusts were tasked with achieving the goal of 'safe and compassionate care'.

The Morecambe Bay Investigation was an inquiry into another scandal-hit Trust, the Furness General Hospital in Cumbria and its maternity unit. The inquiry, chaired by Bill Kirkup, found that there were many failings in the monitoring of the organisation, much like those in the Mid Staffordshire Trust that had been highlighted only a few years prior in the 'Francis Report'. The inquiry found that poor care had possibly contributed to the death of mothers and babies at the unit. The scathing inquiry found that there were poor standards set by the internal investigations and that interventions as far back as 2003 could have had led to changes that would have prevented future deaths (Wise, 2015). The inquiry also discovered that practice had drifted away from expected standards to practice that was unsafe, which was only found out once multiple serious incidents had taken place. The Trust had not shared accessible adverse incident information that revealed the extent of the poor care delivered as it was concerned that it would have an impact on the attainment of foundation trust status.

The inquiry concluded with multiple recommendations for the Trust and for the wider NHS and stated:

What is inexcusable, however, is the repeated failure to examine adverse events properly, to be open and honest with those who suffered, and to learn so as to prevent recurrence. Yet this is what happened consistently over the whole period 2004–12, and each instance represents a significant lapse from the professional duty of NHS staff.

(Kirkup 2015: 183)

It is well established (Dixon-Woods et al., 2014), that the impact of treating staff and clinicians with respect and compassion leads to 'improved patient satisfaction, infection and mortality rates, Care Quality Commission (CQC) ratings and financial performance and lower turnover and absenteeism' (108). Is there a reason why NHS organisations will not then use this approach? The answer may lie in national guidance and the expected slow pace of change, despite a realisation that current practice needs to improve.

The UK systems and processes to review untoward incidents have evolved over the last few decades. The standards of reviewing and providing assurance are set centrally by NHS England, who publish national guidance on a regular basis. The most recent guidance is the Patient Safety Incident Response Framework, first published in 2020 (NHS England, 2022).

When a serious untoward incident (SUI) occurs, NHS organisations are bound by the Patient Safety Incident Response Framework (NHS England, 2022) to provide assurance that organisations have robust systems in place to respond when things go wrong. The expectation is that the organisations have a mechanism to identify issues in the system and learn from them to prevent such harm coming to patients in the future. Sadly, as reported by the British Medical Association in 2018, the processes in existence have led to staff being harmed. It is a sad state of affairs when a process meant to focus on learning has led to blame, shame, and abuse, which in turn, has led to poorer outcomes for patients.

The question we must ask ourselves is 'Why do investigations cause harm to those who delivered care?' As a medical professional and clinician, I have reflected on why things have not gone to plan when my team has delivered care. It is almost always in the context of working in a busy environment and under pressure to complete competing tasks in an unsafe system. However, this does not take away from the fact that care delivered has led to harm, and a fellow human has suffered as a result of care delivered with the best of intentions.

'Second victims', as described by Wu in 2000, are those healthcare professionals who are psychologically or professionally harmed by the unanticipated healthcare error that led to harm being caused to a patient. This view, that professionals are impacted in significant ways, has not led to development of robust support for them within the work environment and certainly not in the NHS. There is little published literature around 'second victims' and the impact on clinicians professionally and personally, but efforts being made by organisations such as Second Victim Support, who support clinicians affected through patient safety incidents, a programme developed in the UK by the Yorkshire Quality and Safety Research Group and the Improvement Academy, are the shoots of what is needed across healthcare settings.

Can the process of providing assurance, allegedly one that sets out to learn from incidents, be inherently unsuitable for identifying learning and making improvements in the care delivered? Kumar et al. (2020) noted in their article about root cause analysis (RCA) in the NHS that it was indeed time for change as the methodology was flawed in that it inherently aims to 'protect institutional reputation'. In their article they noted that it was not the case that incidents occurred as a result of one root cause and that they were usually the result of multiple intertwined systemic issues. Anecdotally, I have seen that the factors that affect an outcome are multifactorial, but organisations were bound to use national guidance and approaches such as RCAs, which directed reviewers to find a 'root cause'. It has been the case that RCAs undertaken in NHS organisations found that an individual or team was responsible for the poor outcomes. This has a profound impact on the individual and the team. In the Trust I work for, the culture and practice many years ago was to 'suspend' staff until an RCA or 'investigation' was completed and 'blame' had been apportioned. Thankfully, this practice has ceased within the organisation as there is an understanding that being open and honest about errors that may have taken place allows staff to think collaboratively of ways to avoid harm from happening again. Overall, there is no doubt that it leads to safer care. However, it did take some time for staff and clinicians to be reassured that being open and transparent was not going subject them to adverse criticism. There needed to be a change in culture and approach that was supported by the organisation's board. That was what happened in the Trust that I work in. The Trust, with committed support of the Chief Executive and Director of Human Resources, developed the Restorative and 'Just Culture' approach within the Trust after dismissals and investigations of staff reached a high in 2015–2016.

The approach was not new as it was noted in many articles by Professor Sidney Dekker, whose book *Just Culture* (2012) lays out the tenets of working within a restorative just culture that underpinned the Trust's approach. The Trust began its journey to become an organisation that embraced Just and Learning Culture (JLC) and over the years has shown the benefits of such an approach to staff and external stakeholders. The Trust uses an evolved version of Just Culture known as Restorative Just Culture (RJC) as described by Dekker. The cultural shift away from asking 'who' was responsible to 'what' went wrong can be a significant contributor to how organisations respond to serious incidents, and it was a new path for us.

In my area of clinical practice, there are examples of how, in the past, staff have been suspended when things have not gone to plan. This has led to numerous instances of staff becoming 'second victims'. There have been instances where staff have been suspended or even dismissed on the basis of versions of events that have later been discredited by employment tribunals, external independent reviews (Kirkup, 2018), or our own internal reviews. The remarks by Dr Kirkup in his independent report into Liverpool Community Health Trust's care were so damaging that the Trust was acquired by another Trust soon after. The report highlights instances where staff were suspended for raising concerns and those who raised grievances were summarily suspended for months without the offer of an explanation or understanding of the impact this would have on their mental and physical wellbeing. Again, as seen with the Morecambe Bay Investigation, a culture of under-reporting, fear when raising concerns, and an acceptance by the board of risks to patient safety in pursuit of FT status had an impact on staff and patient wellbeing.

The significant impact that an uncaring and punitive environment has on the wellbeing of staff and the consequences for patient safety cannot be underestimated. This cultural shift to RJC also underpins the recently published NHS Patient Safety Incident Response Framework (PSIRF) (NHS England, 2022) guidance, which talks about how organisational cultures needs to move to a place of 're-flection and learning' rather than one working to an 'accountability framework'. The PSIRF, which was required to be implemented by all NHS organisations by Autumn 2023, is underpinned by the principles of 'openness, fair accountability, learning and continuous improvement'. NHS organisations were expected to have made arrangements to implement the PSIRF whilst still using the old Serious Incident Framework (NHS England, 2015).

It is hoped that with the implementation of the PSIRF, organisations will move to being more open and honest about errors that have been made by them and their employees, and engage with families and those that they cared for, enabling those conversations about the care their loved ones received.

In our Trust, plans are afoot to move to PSIRF and underpin our review of serious incident using the restorative justice and learning culture approach. Work is already underway, and the way we conduct our reviews has been gradually changing from the investigative process from ten years ago to a more collaborative, listening exercise that identifies the systemic issues at play when things do not go to plan. Over the course of the last three years, we have moved away in the Trust from undertaking RCAs to undertaking learning reviews (LRs). This process is one that is fully understood by the locality Senior Coroner and is underpinned by the principles of openness, honesty, and transparency, so that the review leads to most learning. In order to make the process more robust, we set out to ensure that the emphasis was about learning and feedback. Process mapping exercises undertaken four years ago showed the lack of impact regarding demonstrable learning from RCAs and the need to move to LRs where the team and staff who delivered care were involved in the collaborative review, with families leading the questions being asked. It is now standard practice to have families involved from the very beginning and have a family liaison officer (FLO) make that initial contact and ensure that the family's voice is heard. Any questions raised by the family are then addressed by the review panel in the LR. Readers will no doubt have noted the move away from using the word 'investigation' to using the word 'reviews'. This has had a profound impact on the wellbeing of staff as the notion that the process is punitive is shifting to one where there is genuine acceptance of it being one for learning.

We know from the aviation industry the importance of being open and honest. There is much to learn from the aviation industry about safety and the importance of being open and honest. Legislation allows this for the aviation industry, something that is not available in healthcare. However, the move away from RCAs to LRs that are underpinned by being open, honest, and transparent, although not set out in legislation, will allow a shift in culture. Anecdotally, in our Trust, clinicians who are involved in delivering care are now more likely to engage in the process of learning from serious incidents and deaths than they have been in the past. Our LRs now must include the lead clinician, usually a doctor and the operational and clinical manager so that recommendations are realistic, and feedback is immediate as to what needs to be improved. This approach of getting clinicians involved in making the recommendations and agreeing to deliver the improvements is more likely to lead to improvements in quality and safety. We have now set up an internal learning platform that staff can access to learn about serious incidents, share useful practices across the organisation, and improve outcomes for patients we care for in our services. In order to ensure that the learning from reviews of serious incidents and other safety issues leads to meaningful outcomes, the Trust set up a Trust-wide Strategic Quality Improvement Group that monitors the impact of reviews and the subsequent learning on quality of care.

### Is there a financial argument for improving serious incident reviews?

If the argument that quality and safety of patient care improves with Just Culture has not been bought into by senior leaders, Trust board members, etc., then a further driver for change might be an economic one.

There is ample evidence from published literature about the drivers of change in the NHS. The main drivers for change in the NHS are thought to be political followed by financial. Both these factors have a significant impact on patient experience. The requirement from the government to save money to manage the annual budget of the NHS means that organisations are under more scrutiny and are being pushed to work more efficiently. The NHS efficiency map produced by NHS England, NHS Improvement, and the Healthcare Financial Management Association (HFMA) (HFMA, 2019) talks about the importance of having efficient systems from board to wards so that effective decisions can be made to ensure the best possible outcomes for patients. The report talks about the importance of system efficiency to ensure cost savings are achieved. Clearly, a financial burden on the NHS will have an impact on quality delivered. The report published in January 2022 by the Department of Health and Social Care about introducing a legal cap on money that is spent on litigation on clinical negligence cases, which has seen costs rise significantly from around £582 million in 2006–2007 to over £2 billion in 2020–2021, will be another driver for reducing costs and improving savings. In the Trust I work in, there has been a move towards early resolution, and this might include financial compensation when someone has come to harm. It negates the needs for expensive legal costs to be paid out and it allows families and patients who have come to harm to have resolution of the complaints or claims addressed in a manner that allows them to accept and move on quickly. It frees up valuable time for the organisation to focus on making the necessary improvements in response to the complaints and claims made, a win-win for all involved.

The question is whether there is a financial case for moving away from a punitive and disciplinary process to a supportive and learning process when it comes to managing staff who have been involved in complaints and serious incidents. In their article about the economic impact of implementing restorative justice, Kaur and colleagues (2019) discuss the significant savings an organisation made with the implementation of a restorative culture. The savings are not insignificant at about £2.5 million a year. If there is anyone now arguing that getting it right the first time is not the right approach, there is now an economic argument in favour of getting it right. Calculating the economic cost reduction is not an easy task, but the amount saved by that Trust was 1 per cent of their annual income. It was achieved by a combination of approaches to manging suspensions and disciplinary actions using a restorative approach.

In conclusion, we can hope that there is light at the end of this tunnel of serious incident reviews. At the Royal College of Psychiatrists' Congress in Edinburgh (June 2022), there was overwhelming support for a new process of learning from serious incidents and to do away with RCAs as a tool in mental health care reviews. With the publication of the PSIRF, and the move away from RCAs towards LRs that is underpinned by a restorative justice and learning culture approach, we can hope that organisations begin to listen to the voices of the families and patients who have been harmed inadvertently whilst we endeavour to provide care in a less-than-perfect system. The move towards collaborative reviews, involving families and giving them feedback, can only be a step in the right direction.

## References

British Medical Association. (2018). Fatigue and sleep deprivation. Available from: www.bma. org.uk/advice-and-support/nhs-delivery-and-workforce/creating-a-healthy-workplace/fatigue-and-sleep-deprivation

Dekker, S. W. A. (2012). *Just Culture: Balancing Safety and Accountability* (2nd ed.). Farnham: Ashgate Publishing.

Department of Health and Social Care. (2014). 'Francis Effect' on NHS care one year on from Mid Staffs Inquiry. Available from: www.gov.uk/government/news/francis-effect-on-nhs-care-one-year-on-from-mid-staffs-inquiry

Department of Health and Social Care. (2022). New cap on legal costs to save NHS £500 million. Available from: www.gov.uk/government/news/new-cap-on-legal-costs-to-save-nhs-500-million

Dixon-Woods, M., Baker, R., Charles, K., Dawson, J., Jerzembek, G., Martin, G.,... & West, M. (2014). Culture and behaviour in the English National Health Service: Overview of lessons from a large multimethod study. *BMJ Quality & Safety*, 23(2), 106–115.

Donaldson, L. (2002). An organisation with a memory. *Clinical Medicine*, 2(5), 452–457.

Francis, R. (2013). *Report of the Mid Staffordshire NHS Foundation Trust Public Inquiry: executive summary* (Vol. 947). London: The Stationery Office.

Havens, D. H., & Boroughs, L. (2000). 'To err is human': A report from the Institute of Medicine. *Journal of Pediatric Health Care*, 14(2), 77–80.

Health Financial Management Association. (2019). NHS efficiency map Available from: www.hfma.org.uk/system/files?file=nhs-efficiency-map-updated-january-2017.pdf&sfvrsn=0

Kaur, M., De Boer, R. J., Oates, A., Rafferty, J., & Dekker, S. (2019). Restorative just culture: a study of the practical and economic effects of implementing restorative justice in an NHS Trust. In *MATEC Web of Conferences* (Vol. 273). EDP Sciences.

Kirkup, B., (2015). *The Report of the Morecambe Bay Investigation.* Available from: www.gov.uk/government/publications/morecambe-bay-investigation-report

Kirkup, B. (2018). *Report of the Liverpool Community Health Independent Review.* Available from: www.england.nhs.uk/publication/report-of-the-liverpool-community-health-independent-review

Kumar, S., Kline, R., & Boylin, T. (2020). Root cause analysis in the NHS: Time for change? *British Journal of Hospital Medicine*, 81(4), 1–4.

NHS England. (2015). *Serious Incident Framework: Supporting learning to prevent recurrence.* Available from: www.england.nhs.uk/patientsafety/wp-content/uploads/sites/32/2015/04/serious-incidnt-framwrk-upd2.pdf

NHS England. (2022). Patient Safety Incident Response Framework and supporting guidance. Available from: www.england.nhs.uk/publication/patient-safety-incient-response-framework-and-supporting-guidance

Panagioti, M., Khan, K., Keers, R. N., Abuzour, A., Phipps, D., Kontopantelis, E., & Ashcroft, D. M. (2019). Prevalence, severity, and nature of preventable patient harm across medical care settings: Systematic review and meta-analysis. *BMJ*, 366, 14185.

Wise, J. (2015). Substandard care at 'dysfunctional' Morecambe Bay maternity unit led to unnecessary deaths. *BMJ*, 350, h1221.

World Health Organization. (2019). Patient Safety. Available from: www.who.int/news-room/fact-sheets/detail/patient-safety

Wu, A. W. (2000). Medical error: The second victim. The doctor who makes the mistake needs help too. *BMJ*, 320(7237), 726–727.

# 18 The coroner's inquest and attendance at an inquest hearing

*Louise Swarbrick*

This chapter focuses largely on the experience of professionals working in health and social care professions, due to the experience of the author; however, the principles of presenting in court are largely transferable, as is the anxiety evoked by this.

A primary aim of public service workers and professions is to protect others from unnecessary harm; indeed, many have a *duty of care* to prevent harm. Professionals working in statutory agencies with adults with care and support needs have a fundamental task to provide care and achieve the best outcome for the person. Even exceptional care cannot prevent deaths by natural causes. For any practitioner, facing an inquest hearing can be anxiety provoking, disconcerting, and somewhat confusing, and may leave the practitioner feeling criticised, blamed, or under the spotlight. The aim of this chapter is to offer a pragmatic overview of the role of the coroner's inquest, planning for attendance at an inquest hearing, what happens during the hearing, and what to expect following the delivery of a verdict. Coroners serve as impartial judicial officers and specialise in examining specific causes of death. The role of the coroner is to investigate deaths if they have reason to suspect that the death was violent or unnatural, the cause of death is unknown, or the deceased died whilst in state detention (Courts and Tribunals Judiciary, 2024). Coroners are usually lawyers or doctors funded by the local authority, subject to a set of particular rules, who seek to establish facts in order to identify a cause of death (Cave, 2012).

Griffith and Tengnah (2023) recognise that the prospect of having to appear in court can be intimidating as the process is formalised and tends to be steeped in tradition, and the associated language, rules, and custom will be unfamiliar to many. Increased awareness of what is expected before, during, and after an inquest equips professionals to prepare for and make a meaningful contribution to this process.

## The voice of experience

Laura (a nurse) (pseudonym) was called to produce a witness statement for the coroner for a death in a mental health hospital setting whereby a patient was found with a ligature tied; tragically, the patient died following a period of acute hospital treatment for injuries sustained. Laura, who had been a witness as part of a local

DOI: 10.4324/9781003286240-23

investigation, had provided witness statements, and had been interviewed as part of this process, describes the experience of being identified by the coroner as a key witness in an inquest. The account below exemplifies that of many when they are called to give witness in a coroners' court.

*I felt like nothing had prepared me for the notification from the coroner, even when it is expected as part of the process following a death of this nature. I noticed how I was responding to certain situations at work with caution, trying to avoid or prevent this happening again to anyone else I was working with. I received support from my line manager to talk through this in clinical supervision, alongside accessing organisational support via a counselling service for a one-off session; this helped particularly with ongoing management of people at high risk of suicide. I found the legal team who work on behalf of the NHS Trust I was employed by extremely helpful in navigating the process of the coroner and what to expect, and providing assistance with writing the witness statement.*

*I was concerned about having to attend court. I had never had to give a witness statement in court for someone I had been working so closely with; having to face the family and bear witness to their grief was also on my mind. I felt so guilty despite knowing I was not to blame, I also felt guilty for feeling those feelings too when there was a family experiencing the loss of a loved one. I suppose when you work so closely to develop a therapeutic relationship with someone, there is an element of grief and loss in there for the nurse/patient relationship. There was for me. I worried my practice would come under scrutiny and I would have to face consequences. I worried I had let the family and the deceased down too.*

*The preparation by the legal team in meetings prior to the hearing, the support from my line manager and having someone in court – in this instance, the solicitor for the NHS Trust I was employed by – was invaluable. I was told the hearing could last a number of days; there were several key witnesses and there would be a jury. I was told this was because of the complexities of the case. I felt like I was facing trial; however, the solicitor provided reassurances and explained the role of the coroner and the inquisitorial hearing procedure to me. I was there to relay a factual account of my professional involvement, and my written statement would need to reflect the same. The solicitor attended pre-inquest hearings on behalf of the organisation I worked for; she relayed my witness statement and met with me twice before the inquest hearing date. I had the opportunity to ask questions and review my statement, and to be briefed on how the hearing would be conducted.*

*The solicitor took time in the morning to meet with me for a coffee before court; this allayed my fears and, on reflection, it was important to have some thinking time and de-brief before the hearing. I was glad to have someone in the court room who had become familiar to me; I would've requested my line manager to attend with me if the solicitor hadn't. I entered court, acknowledged the family in a polite, respectful, and courteous manner. I sat in the viewing gallery until I was called to the stand. I was told beforehand I would need to take an oath, and I opted for a non-religious version; there are different versions available for individual preferences. I relayed my statement in a professional and concise way to the court, addressing the judge and jury and then any witnesses who asked questions of me, including the solicitor on behalf of the family. If I wasn't sure of the answer or did not feel I was the best suited witness to give a response, I let the judge know.*

Laura (pseudonym), registered nurse

A coronial investigation is a fact-finding inquiry limited to establishing who has died and when, and where and how the death occurred. A coroner's inquest is inquisitorial in principle and does not seek to establish matters of blame or liability (Griffith, 2017), in contrast to the adversarial principles followed in criminal courts, whereby the prosecution and defence present cases for and against and usually result in a guilty not-guilty verdict. The inquest is very different to a criminal trial and is centred around a process of investigation, led by the coroner and the coroner's officers, rather than apportioning blame (Cave, 2012). Nonetheless, the inquest is a public investigation which can lead to criticism of individuals or organisations, which can have further ramifications.

Certain deaths necessitate an inquest led by a coroner's investigation, particularly in cases of violent or unnatural deaths, sudden deaths of unknown cause, or deaths in police, prison, or state custody or care. The inquest is initiated promptly after the death, to record it, identify the deceased, and authorise a burial or cremation as soon as possible, for the sake of the family who may be traumatised by events (Kirton-Darling, 2022).

Following the opening of an inquest, it may be adjourned until other investigations, including serious investigation reports, are completed. The length of adjournment is at the coroner's discretion, potentially prolonged for complex cases. Pre-inquest hearings or reviews may be conducted before the inquest. Coroner's officers, acting under the direction of the coroner, receive death reports, conduct inquiries, and liaise with bereaved families, police, doctors, and witnesses.

To aid the coroner's inquiry, the coroner may seek details including reports and local policies or protocols related to the individual's care and management before their death. The coroner, determining via necessary evidence and its sources, will request information from anyone whom they identify as key witnesses. In the inquest, the coroner, having gathered all the relevant data, will decide which witnesses they wish to call on to attend court. It is at the coroner's discretion to decide upon the attendance of witnesses at the inquest, and if a witness is unable to attend, they must provide reasons to the coroner. There are timeframes and deadlines that need to be met during this process, and organisations can have financial penalties imposed upon them if these timeframes are not met.

When a person is in the care of the state – in a hospital or care or custodial setting, for example – and their death is identified as not arising from natural causes, an 'article 2 inquest' is requested by the investigating coroner. Article 2 refers to the European Convention of Human Rights, whereby the state's responsibility for a person's life is in question (Human Rights Act, 1998). These investigations can be more extensive and involve a detailed examination to determine if any systemic issues or state agents contributed to the death, ensuring the right to life under article 2. Although similar processes to a non-article 2 inquest, the critical language used, criticisms of individuals through acts of omission or negligent practice identified, and lessons learned for organisations are commonplace (Peate, 2023). In some cases, referrals are made for criminal proceedings or for fitness to practise to regulatory bodies such as the Nursing and Midwifery Council (2018) or the General Medical Council (2024).

Cave (2012) highlights that the hearing could be at a time where concurrent investigations are ongoing and sensitive discussions with the family of the deceased are continuing. There may be organisational priorities to follow, internal reporting and investigation procedures, and the need to manage the risk of reputational damage. Open, honest, and transparent approaches throughout all steps in the process leading up to, during and after the hearing are of utmost importance and uphold legal, ethical, and practical guidance relating to professional standards and conduct (Griffith, 2017).

The National Quality Board (2018) produced guidance relating to working with bereaved families and their carers. Although this guidance was written for the benefit of NHS trusts, the messages within this document refer to a compassionate, open, and honest approach when communicating with families and carers in what can be extremely difficult and emotive periods following the death of a loved one. Section 38 of the Care Act (2014) places emphasis on health and social care professionals having a duty of candour (see Chapters 3 and 4). This requires providers to be open and transparent with individuals and their families when things go wrong. In relation to a coroner's inquest, this may be via investigations to provide lessons learned, the professional maintaining integrity, professionalism, and transparency when providing witness statements and testimonies, and offering an apology.

Writing a statement for an inquest may come some time after the event has occurred, using previous records held, and having the opportunity to access these for review, in order to provide a factual recollection is necessary. This can be a daunting task, one that is likely to require some guidance (Dean, 2021). Laura was able to seek support from her employer (the NHS), and even organisations that do not have their own legal team are well advised to access legal services before writing their statement preparing for court. Many professional organisations offer this – for example, the Royal College of Nursing.

A review of the records is advised to enable a comprehensive account of involvement with a case. When writing a witness statement for the coroner as a professional, specific details will be included about the person's condition, any health diagnoses or symptoms, and the care and treatment or management plans used.

Peate (2023) advises that a factual and objective tone is required, focusing on an accurate account of the individual's professional involvement; speculation or conjecture should be actively avoided. Furthermore, Peate (2023) states that if a professional is struggling to recall events and the information is not held within the records to support what actions were taken, describing standard practice and what would usually occur in situations should be included, ensuring that there is reference to what is a factual account based on information held in records, what is from recollection, and what is standard practice. It is important to stay mindful of the language used within the report, avoiding emotive language, jargon, and complicated terminology, alongside paying attention to any references to protected characteristics or personal traits of the deceased or their family members.

The statement should be written as concisely as possible, so that a lay person could understand what is presented within it. It would be advisable to keep a copy of the statement; it is a legal document, one that could be needed later. If there are any questions about professional standards or conduct, the statement could be shared with staff representatives from a union or legal representative for checking before this is submitted. Local policies and procedures within organisations may have policies that are required to be adhered to, which should also be consulted.

Once the statement has been prepared, checked, and submitted within the time-frame required, the coroner will decide whether the person making the statement is required in the hearing as a key witness.

**Tips for attending court as a key witness (NHS Resolution, 2020):**

- Consider taking a copy of your statement and reading this prior to the hearing. You are able to take a copy with you, and there will also be a copy of this available for you at the courtroom.
- Arrive early on the day – at least half an hour prior to the inquest commencing.
- Dress appropriately, remembering that court is a formal process. Dress as though you were attending an interview, avoiding bright colours.
- The oath, whether you have opted for a religious or non-religious version, is a declaration of speaking the truth. To do otherwise could be contempt of court, which may result in criminal prosecution.
- Speak slowly, clearly, and concisely.
- Give a full, honest, and objective accounts to the questions asked. Remain factual, avoiding using subjective language.
- Address your answers to the coroner or the person asking the questions.
- If asked a question and you are not sure you understand its meaning, ask the coroner or the person asking the question to repeat it or ask for further clarity.

- If you are unable to answer the question because you do not know the answer, let the court know you do not know.
- If you feel the question would be best answered by another key witness, let the coroner know.

Following the hearing, it is advisable to seek support for debrief, organisational support for any media interest that may occur, legal assistance and staff-side support for any potential criminal investigations. The outcome may result in further exploration of events leading up to the death, such as procedural changes or recommendations for organisations and systems to improve their ways of working (Ministry of Justice, 2013). The coroner can also write a report to prevent future deaths (Coroners and Justice Act, 2009). In support of promoting just cultures, leaders supporting staff members during inquest hearings could consider adopting a compassionate leadership response.

In some cases, there may be identification of gross misconduct by individuals uncovered by the coroner's review; this could result in disciplinary action or fitness to practise proceedings (see Chapter 13) being instigated or local human resources policies for performance management actioned. It is important to consider, if not earlier identified and actioned in any local incident reviews, contact with families or carers of the deceased to offer apologies.

Let's return to 'Laura' who has a word of advice for us:

*My advice would be for anyone in a professional capacity attending an inquest to reach out for help and advice, take time to go through the process once the witness statement request lands in your inbox. Having time, space, and support to process how I felt before the hearing enabled me to convey my statement in a calm and professional manner in court. Afterwards, I was informed of the verdict of death by misadventure via a narrative verdict by the solicitor in a telephone call, which later followed in an email. There were some lessons learned for the organisation, and I am aware these have been implemented locally. This doesn't negate the loss of life, I recognise that.*

## Conclusion

Inquests, as intimidating as they may be, are a necessary legal process to establish the cause of death. With greater emphasis on preparedness and highlighting what to expect, it is hoped that professionals may be able to approach these with less worry and greater awareness of the processes dictated by court hearings, enabling them to access the support needed to do so.

This chapter has attempted to provide some background to the processes and to provide some insight into the process.

# References

Care Act. (2014). c.23. (2015). Available from: www.legislation.gov.uk/ukpga/2014/23/contents/enacted

Cave, T. (2012). Calling in the coroner: The investigation process. *Journal of Nursing & Residential Care*, 14 (9).

Coroners and Justice Act. (2009). c. 25. Available from: www.legislation.gov.uk/ukpga/2009/25/contents

Courts and Tribunals Judiciary (2024). Coroners' Courts. Available from: www.judiciary.uk/courts-and-tribunals/coroners-courts

Dean, E. (2021). Coroner's inquests: What you need to know if you are asked to give evidence. *Nursing Standard*, 36(4), 26–28.

General Medical Council. (2024). *Good Medical Practice: professional standards.* Available from: www.gmc-uk.org/professional-standards/professional-standards-for-doctors/good-medical-practice

Griffith, R., & Tengnah, C. (2023). Principles of good evidence giving. *British Journal of Community Nursing*, 10(11), 542–544.

Griffith, R. (2017). Professionalism in practice: The coroner's court. *British Journal of Community Nursing*, 22(1), 685–687.

Human Rights Act. (1998). c.42. Available from: www.legislation.gov.uk/ukpga/1998/42

Kirton-Darling, E. (2022). Dignity, the Family and the Body. In *Death, Family and the Law.* Bristol: Bristol University Press.

Ministry of Justice. (2013). *The Coroners Investigations Regulations.* SI 2013/1629.

National Quality Board. (2018). *National Guidance on Learning from Deaths.* Available from: www.england.nhs.uk/wp-content/uploads/2017/03/nqb-national-guidance-learning-from-deaths.pdf

NHS Resolution. (2020). *Inquests: A guide for health providers. Supporting staff to prepare for an inquest.* Available from: https://resolution.nhs.uk/wp-content/uploads/2020/03/Inquests-films-and-guide.pdf

Nursing and Midwifery Council (2018). *The Code: Professional Standards of practice and behaviour for nurses, midwives and nursing associates.* Available from: www.nmc.org.uk/standards/code

Peate, I. (2023) Coping with investigations and statement writing. *British Journal of Healthcare Assistants*, 17(10), 380–384.

# 19 Closing the loop

## Creating learning from the incident

*Kim Bennett and Panchu Xavier*

'The phrase "lessons will be learned" rings hollow when history shows us that so often in the NHS, they simply are not' (Titcombe and Montgomery, 2022). James Titcombe was writing in response to the much-awaited Final Ockenden report on the findings of the review into maternity services at Shrewsbury and Telford NHS Trust, published in March 2022 (Department of Health, 2022). Having experienced the personal loss of his baby son at another NHS Trust in 2008, James did not fully learn of the circumstances of his son's death until 2015 after the publication of an investigation into maternity services. The review of Morecambe Bay maternity services also identified failures at every level within the healthcare system (Department of Health, 2015).

James Titcombe's words, and those of Nadine Montgomery quoted within the same 2022 article, are heartfelt and outline what they term 'common themes' in the failure to make the changes necessary to improve safety in maternity services. This failure to learn lessons was reinforced by the findings of the independent investigation into maternity and neonatal services in East Kent, in October 2022, which rather than make recommendations, as previous reports have without any changes taking place, identified areas for action. These areas for action are that the NHS becomes better at identifying poorly performing services, at providing care with kindness and compassion, at teamworking with a shared aim, and at responding to challenges with honesty (Kirkup, 2022).

There have previously been many reviews and reports into significant events within health and social services, each with major recommendations and the perhaps now discredited phrase 'lessons will be learnt' accompanying their publication. It is not unreasonable to ask if lessons were to have been learnt, why changes have not been incorporated into systems and practice to prevent the recurrence of tragic circumstances such as those experienced by the patients and families across the UK.

This chapter will review some of the factors that impact the apparent difficulties health and social care have faced in implementing lessons learnt from investigations that are carried out. We will consider how to overcome the mismatch between knowledge and insight gained from incident reviews and the transfer of such insight into practice.

DOI: 10.4324/9781003286240-24

We also offer our own review and guidance on the use of more commonly known practical methodologies to maximise the effectiveness of sharing of learning with particular reference to those suggested in the Patient Safety Incident Response Framework (PSIRF) toolkit (Department of Health, 2020).

## Background

'With ... complexity comes an inevitable risk that at times things will go wrong' (Department of Health, 2000: 6). Formerly, the absence of adverse incidents would have been considered the ultimate goal of a successful organisation – what Hollnagel describes as a Safety I approach. A Safety II perspective conversely considers if an organisation has an in-built ability to function as required or if its systems maximise outcomes that are acceptable (Hollnagel, 2022). To achieve this, and successfully learn, we need to review when things have not gone as planned but equally review when success has been achieved. This is a quantum leap from patient safety review methodologies based on seeking a single root cause or, more commonly, identifying where an individual member of staff went wrong. Along with other high-risk industries, it is widely recognised that when things go wrong in healthcare, it is not usually an individual's error; rather, incidents arise from the complexities of the system and environment in which they are working (NHS Improvement, 2018).

Instead, we should seek to establish the circumstances of why the actions of the individual under investigation made sense to them at the time. In our experience, recommendations arising from patient safety reviews rarely note a requirement for any organisational-level actions, focusing solely on the sharp end of Trust activity and on the individual practitioners or team (Dekker, 2012; Dekker et al., 2022).

This forms the basis of the approach to patient safety reviews in PSIRF which suggests that an organisation needs to be culturally ready for this approach to be able to undertake any investigation in a meaningful way and also to assimilate learning and utilise this to promote safety.

## Cultures which promote learning

We have all heard the saying 'Culture eats strategy for breakfast' (Guley & Reznik, 2019). The culture of an organisation is driven by the senior management, and in the NHS most organisations reportedly have a 'blame culture'. However, an alternative to this has been suggested, and there is much in the published literature about the benefits of a 'just culture'. The first discussions about the need for a 'just culture' came from the work of James Reason in his book *Managing the Risks of Organizational Accidents*, published in 1997. He argued that to have a safety culture in an organisation, you needed to have a 'just culture' in place. This concept was noted by David Marx, who in his publication on 'Patient Safety and Just Culture' in 2001, elaborates on the impact that just culture can have on healthcare systems in transfusion safety. It was imperative that individuals felt it was safe to raise concerns that would lead to better learning and outcomes for patients. It was noted that disciplining staff who had made honest mistakes did little to improve safety in the system and this led to thinking in academia around 'Just Culture' and the impact it could have in healthcare systems.

Von Thaden et al. (2006) discussed the perception of just culture in healthcare and how organisations that had adopted just culture had improved patient safety. This was further supported by Khatri et al. (2009) in their paper on moving from a blame culture to a just culture in healthcare. They wrote about how a blame culture was more likely in organisations that had hierarchical, compliance-based management systems in place as opposed to those that had a collaborative approach with employees and were more likely to have a just culture approach. So, the question is why wouldn't we have Just Culture in healthcare organisations? The answer sadly lies in national guidance for NHS organisations in the United Kingdom and in similar guidance elsewhere, rooted in legal adversarial processes surrounding litigation with regard to harm.

The move away from this process is welcomed in the most recent NHS guidance. The Patient Safety Incident Response Framework (NHS England, 2020) asks that NHS and healthcare providers move away from the processes set out in the previous guidance, the Serious Incident Framework (NHS England, 2015b), to one that is open, honest, and collaborative with families and patients who have been harmed.

Our Trust transitioned into this in 2023, and has been a pioneer in 'Just and Learning Culture', which has been embedded in human resources (HR) processes for many years. The public website of Mersey Care NHS Foundation Trust (2022) gives you access to modules that any organisation can utilise to begin their journey of the Just and Learning Culture (JLC) process. They refer to the 4-Step process that uses a checklist to ensure that staff are supported during the HR process. The JLC process underpins the trust's Adverse Incident Management Policy 2022. This allows staff to talk openly about the incident, safe in the knowledge that the trust's JLC approach is embedded in the processes of the policy. The shift away from punitive processes to one that is supportive and collaborative has led to improved staff satisfaction results for the trust. There is evidence that there is an upward trajectory in the reporting of incidents, a sign of a healthy reporting culture. Continuing review is needed to monitor the impact on harm levels and confirm a true safety culture.

### Using knowledge and sharing learning – learning processes in action

Whilst culture and leadership can create the environment necessary for an organisation to become safe, there will need to be systems and processes in place to respond to and allow for investigation, or review, of events. We have already noted how a positive restorative culture can benefit those involved in an incident and allow for learning to be maximised. This paradigm still requires a means to fully explore that learning. Whether they have negative or positive outcomes, events need to be fully understood and the circumstances involved appreciated to allow for restorative processes to take place. Organisations must have arrangements in place for this mechanism to inform improvement in culture, practice, and delivery of services going forward.

Within the original PSIRF, several devices are outlined to respond to patient safety incidents (Department of Health, 2020) and derive findings from such events. It should be acknowledged that the wider complexities involved in a modern healthcare system can provide both drivers and blocks to accessing this insight and improvement on both a personal professional and broader health economy basis. Peerally et al. (2017) have rightly criticised the former focus on the production of a serious incident report as the desired end product of an investigation process rather than 'the beginning of the learning cycle'. We would agree with this criticism but also suggest that learning actually starts within the information-gathering phase, with the active involvement of those involved.

Clearly, the methodology selected needs to 'fit' the circumstances of the particular event. Tools can and should offer the potential opportunities for learning to take place throughout the process of investigation itself to maximise reflection, and the extraction of data, knowledge, and insight. Further, tools may be used in combination where learning can significantly extend beyond an immediate clinical team or service.

To appreciate the usefulness of the various tools described by PSIRF and assist in selection, we have compiled the following summaries of the significant techniques suggested.

Our first summary is of the features of 'hot debriefing'. This term is used to describe a debriefing carried out as close to the incident as possible and distinguishes this from a 'cold' debrief which may take place sometime later incorporating factual data such as downloads of oral or videotape recordings (Hale et al., 2020).

Retrospective case note reviews differ from audits due to the feature of judgement on the part of the reviewer. Royal Colleges have established standardised methodology for case note review in the structured judgement review for review of mortality cases. We have utilised an adapted version of the Royal College of Psychiatrists model within our own organisation to ensure that initial screening captures patients for review across the broad range of mental and physical health services provided. Cases are considered within a weekly mortality multidisciplinary team format to ensure probity and findings are further shared with clinical and governance teams.

AARs mirror a process we have been utilising within our own organisation for the last couple of years. We have been undertaking team-based learning review meetings as part of our serious incident investigation process. As an integral part of information gathering for reviewers, we have gathered the key relevant stakeholders in a joint meeting (both face-to-face and virtually) to explore the circumstances and background of an incident. This allows for an inductive process to establish learning following an incident or event where staff are included and involved to contribute to this. As with AARs, this does require careful facilitation to ensure balance and psychological safety of all.

*Table 19.1* Hot debrief

| Hot debrief | |
|---|---|
| **Description** | Collaborative discussion immediately following an incident or event provided as an opportunity for individuals or teams involved in the incident or event. |
| **Background** | Much of the work on the value of hot debriefing has come from the hyper-acute fields of resuscitation and trauma medicine. |
| **Applicability** | One of the promptest means for promoting learning following a significant event, provided immediately after the event with immediate learning opportunity. |
| **Benefits** | <ul><li>can be used to offer support to staff, ensuring the welfare of those present</li><li>acknowledges that personnel involved or affected by an incident may experience their own psychological impact</li><li>gives an opportunity for self-reflection</li><li>provides an immediate opportunity to improve by sharing successes and challenges experienced by both individuals and teams involved</li><li>can be achieved quickly and allows for staff to return to duties</li></ul> |
| **Limitations** | <ul><li>may not always feel feasible in high-flow/intensity healthcare settings</li><li>requires a physical space for completion due to time restrictions, may not allow for all views and perspectives to be explored</li><li>requires awareness of team dynamics and emotions involved</li><li>may also require a facilitator with technical knowledge</li><li>may be difficult to capture all perspectives and utilise these if not formally documented</li><li>there is no standardised framework or approach to ensure effectiveness</li></ul> |

Table 19.2 Case record/note review

*Case record/note review*

| | |
|---|---|
| **Description** | Review of the medical records of an individual carried out by a trained reviewer following initial screening to meet set criteria. |
| **Background** | Utilised within healthcare on an informal basis for many years but of increased prominence in the USA from the 1970s due to increased litigation costs. |
| **Applicability** | Case note reviews can be carried out for any healthcare discipline. Reviews are usually retrospective but may be contemporaneous. For the most-used structured judgement review methodologies, there is an initial screening to identify individuals for case note review and then a review framework that the reviewer follows. |
| **Benefits** | <ul><li>can be used to identify adverse events</li><li>allows for qualitative review of clinical records for alignment against known data</li><li>can be used to focus on specific elements within the clinical process or cohorts of patients</li><li>allows for good care to be recorded as well as where care has not gone as planned</li><li>avoidability judgements can be based on the complete clinical picture within the notes</li><li>internal reviewers may have an awareness of the systemic context of an organisation</li></ul> |
| **Limitations** | <ul><li>potentially time-consuming – both for initial screening and case note review</li><li>can be subject to outcome and hindsight bias</li><li>inter-reviewer variability</li><li>possibility of equivocation where judgements are not sufficiently specific</li><li>can be incorrectly used to generalise on features</li><li>by their nature, only details included in the case notes can be known</li><li>dependent on the quality and content of the case record</li><li>methodology may not be standardised</li></ul> |

*Table 19.3* After-action review

*After-action review (AAR)*

| | |
|---|---|
| **Description** | A structured, facilitated discussion on an incident or event to identify a group's strengths, weaknesses, and areas for improvement by understanding the expectations and perspectives of all those involved and capturing learning to share more widely. |
| **Background** | Developed with the USA military to enable review of military action to ensure that reflections of staff involved were captured, to improve team capability, and to seek solutions and improvement suggestions. |
| **Applicability** | Although drawn from the military setting, akin to 'cold debrief', this method is applicable across healthcare settings. |
| **Benefits** | • allows analysis of event – whether roles were understood, and goals achieved in the way intended<br>• allows participants to share their personal experience and all perspectives welcomed<br>• use of a trained independent facilitator promotes psychological safety<br>• allows for analysis of outcomes and future planning<br>• improvements can be carried forward by the team itself with specified follow-up actions<br>• can be time limited to a maximum of two hours<br>• could be carried out remotely (although face-to-face preferred) |
| **Limitations** | • requires planning to organise<br>• requires an independent facilitator and a note taker to capture the discussion<br>• if delayed, there is a possibility of memory modification amongst participants<br>• needs careful facilitation to avoid blaming – ground rules for discussion needed<br>• to fully realise the benefits, requires participation and commitment of all relevant personnel |

*Table 19.4* Safety huddle

| Safety huddle | |
|---|---|
| **Description** | A short multi-disciplinary (usually) team meeting to brief team members on a specific risk or potential harm for a cohort of patients. |
| **Background** | Huddles to promote team working and encourage focus have a background in manufacturing and retail where there may be an associated productivity or marketing target. |
| **Applicability** | Huddles can take place within any healthcare setting and may be single or multi-disciplinary. Reactive huddles may take place in response to an incident or event that has already occurred. Proactive huddles may seek to pre-empt or prevent patient safety events. |
| **Benefits** | • huddles can provide an opportunity for an intense focus on a particular safety matter<br>• team members' awareness of the issue is enhanced<br>• a huddle can support collective consideration of solutions in the real-world setting<br>• the huddle is an opportunity to create and sustain psychological safety<br>• the huddle allows a team to share data and celebrate success |
| **Limitations** | • single-discipline safety huddles may not be sufficient to address a particular concern<br>• there needs to be a commitment to attendance within a team and to leadership of the huddle<br>• huddles are intended to be brief and must be strongly led to maintain time frames<br>• huddles are not intended as a patient handover<br>• there is no standardised approach to safety huddles or measuring their effectiveness |

*Table 19.5* Clinical audit

| *Clinical audit* | | |
|---|---|---|
| **Description** | Audit is a quality improvement cycle where the effectiveness of healthcare provision is measured against an agreed standard. This allows for action to follow to ensure that healthcare delivered more closely matches the standard. (Healthcare Quality Improvement Partnership (2012)). | |
| **Background** | Clinical audit purportedly emanates from work completed by Nightingale in the Crimean War. Further seminal work was completed by Codman in the early twentieth century on outcomes from surgery. Many industries utilise audit mechanisms to provide assurance of compliance. | |
| **Applicability** | Audit against agreed standards can take place throughout all spheres of healthcare. | |
| **Benefits** | | **Limitations** |
| • useful for feedback on how an improvement has impacted | | • audit can mistakenly be viewed as an outcome itself |
| • allows for the cycle to operate leading to continuous improvement of outcomes | | • standard statements require clarification to ensure that audits are asking the right questions and reflect current practice |
| • can provide an opportunity for education and training | | • sampling methodology needs consideration to provide reliable information and avoid bias |
| • allows a team to work together in a supportive environment alongside patients | | • audit needs to be acknowledged by senior management to allow changes to follow |
| • clinicians can be supported with data management by audit specialists | | • patient involvement in the process is desirable but will need consideration to make this meaningful and follows ethical practice |

Safety huddles are a common feature in many healthcare settings, usually on a proactive basis (NHS England, 2015a). Reactive huddles could be a useful tool to allow sharing, but consideration would need to be given to how content discussed in the huddle could be captured and reported on. Much of the literature suggests that multi-disciplinary huddles work best allowing for a broader perspective. This requires commitment for attendance from all professional groups and can be maximised by ensuring that job planning includes this element of work.

In our view, the techniques outlined above allow for learning to take place for those directly involved – learning could be said to take place in action. Whilst the national work to introduce PSIRF is ongoing, organisations must consider how to practically allow learning to be utilised from reviews currently being undertaken and implement measures that lead to improvements in systems and practice. This is set against the operational constraints post-Covid-19 and ongoing recruitment and financial limitations. Traditional methods such as newsletters, bulletins, and clinical meetings may be of some value in the physical sharing of learning identified from patient safety incident reviews. Organisations need to work on identifying how using modern technologies and other platforms can help to achieve this. To actually implement change on a systemic level requires understanding and mechanisms to allow for improvement measures to be successful. This is the focus of the next part of our chapter.

### How does an organisation learn from serious incidents?

In their work on organisational learning, Wang and Ahmed (2003) noted the five areas for organisation learning: 'focus on collectivity of individual learning; process or system; culture or metaphor; knowledge management; and continuous improvement'. Clinicians will learn after an incident, but the question remains: does the organisation learn? There is evidence from the literature (Ikehara, 1999) that shows that organisations do not necessarily learn when their staff learn. However, it is important that staff enquire and show a willingness to learn when care has not gone to plan.

A move away from being a punitive process to a supportive one, once things have not gone to plan and caused unintended harm to patients, it is imperative for organisations to learn from this so that harm is not caused again. There is evidence that the culture of the organisation is one important aspect that lends itself to allowing its staff psychological safe spaces to learn and be open and honest about things that have not gone to plan. There must be an understanding of why psychological safety is important in an organisation that wants to become a learning organisation. In her seminal work on psychological safety, Professor Amy Edmondson (1999) speaks about psychological safety being the ability of individuals in organisations to engage in risk-taking interpersonal behaviours that allow them to share their views and fears without retribution or ridicule. In her interview with the Institute for Healthcare Management in 2021 (available on YouTube), Professor Edmonson talks about the four critical outcomes of psychological safety. They are learning, risk management, innovation, and job satisfaction. Learning refers to the learning of the individual and the teams they work in and organisational learning. The ability to ask for help safely allows things to be done more safely. This is turn leads to better risk management by making decisions in a safer manner. Innovation as a result of being allowed to think of new ways of doing things, sharing their thoughts and views without fear of ridicule, is very important and all this leads to job satisfaction. All in all, psychological safety is good for those working in organisation and better for the organisation as well.

So, how do NHS organisations learn from serious incidents? The PSIRF talks about learning and how it needs to be embedded in organisations. The Department of Health white paper 'An organisation with a memory' (Donaldson, 2002) expected NHS organisations to collect data around incidents and learn from it. As a result, multiple national reporting systems were set up and the National Patient Safety Agency (NPSA) was established in 2001. The agency developed the National Reporting and Learning System (NRLS) in 2003. There is evidence (Anderson and Kodate, 2015) that systematic data around incidents can lead to improved patient outcomes and quality of services.

All NHS organisations have internal reporting mechanisms to collect incident data, and this is then analysed to provide assurance to commissioners. However, the methodology used to provide assurance as described in the NHS Serious Incident Framework (NHS England, 2015b) asked organisations to use root cause analysis (RCAs) as its methodology for undertaking investigations into serious incidents. A move away from this was recommended in the Patient Safety Incident Response Framework (Department of Health, 2020) and suggested the use of learning reviews that allow collaborative approaches that involve families and those who were harmed during the episode of care. Our trust, as is the case with many other NHS organisations, is moving towards this approach which is underpinned by a Just and Learning Culture approach, where there is emphasis on psychological safety. The preliminary feedback is that clinicians find these processes more engaging, and service user and patient feedback is that they feel listened to. The trust has developed systems and processes that allow immediate feedback through its 72-hour review process (an immediate learning session that the clinical teams are expected to undertake) to identify learning and share this with other teams. If there has been a death, then an additional process of a screening of the clinical case using the processes set out by the Royal College of Psychiatrists allows a rapid review of care and identification of those cases that need a further structure judgement review (SJR). The SJR process involves senior clinicians to review clinical notes using a structured process and then give feedback to teams about the quality of care. We found that most of the care delivered was good or excellent. If poor care was identified, then an escalation of the review to a learning review is an available next step. Teams are engaged in receiving the positive feedback about good-quality care and are equally engaged in improvements that need to be made. All this is done in a timeframe where the incidents or deaths are still fresh in the minds of the clinicians that delivered care. Such an approach is what most organisations use since the move to the PSIRF in 2023 – the light at the end of the tunnel.

# References

Anderson, J. E., & Kodate, N. (2015). Learning from patient safety incidents in incident review meetings: Organisational factors and indicators of analytic process effectiveness. *Safety Science*, 80, 105–114.

Dekker, S. (2012). *Just Culture: Balancing Safety and Accountability* (2nd ed.). London: CRC Press.

Dekker, S., Oates, A., & Rafferty, J. (eds). (2022). *Restorative Just Culture in Practice: Implementation and Evaluation.* New York: Routledge.

Department of Health. (2000). *An organisation with a memory – Report of an expert group on learning from adverse events in the NHS.* Available from: https://webarchive.nation-alarchives.gov.uk/ukgwa/20130107105354/http://dh.gov.uk/prod_consum_dh/groups/dh_digitalassets/@dh/@en/documents/digitalasset/dh_4065086.pdf

Department of Health. (2015) *The report of the Morecambe Bay Investigation.* Available from: https://assets.publishing.service.gov.uk/government/uploads/system/uploads/attachment_data/file/408480/47487_MBI_Accessible_v0.1.pdf

Department of Health. (2020). *Patient Safety Incident Response Framework 2020: An introductory framework for implementation by nationally appointed early adopters.* Available from: www.england.nhs.uk/wp-content/uploads/2020/08/200312_Introductory_version_of_Patient_Safety_Incident_Response_Framework_FINAL.pdf

Department of Health. (2022). *Ockenden Report – Final: Findings. Conclusions and Essential Actions from the independent Review of Maternity Services at The Shrewsbury and Telford Hospital NHS Trust.* Available from: https://assets.publishing.service.gov.uk/government/uploads/system/uploads/attachment_data/file/1064302/Final-Ockenden-Report-web-accessible.pdf

Donaldson, L. (2002). An organisation with a memory. *Clinical Medicine*, 2(5), 452.

Edmondson, A. C. (1999). Psychological safety and learning behaviour in work teams. *Administrative Science Quarterly,* 44, 350–383

Edmondson A. C. (2021). Why is psychological safety so important in health care? Institute for Healthcare Improvement. YouTube. Available from: www.youtube.com/watch?v=LF1253YhEc8

Guley, G., Reznik, T. (2019). Culture Eats Strategy for Breakfast and Transformation for Lunch. *The Jabian Journal*, 62–65.

Hale, S., Parker, M., Cupido, C., & Kam, A. (2020). Applications of Post resuscitation Debriefing Frameworks in Emergency Settings: A Systematic Review. *AEM Education and Training*, 4(3), 223–230.

Healthcare Quality Improvement Partnership. (2012). *Clinical Audit: A Manual for Lay Members of the Clinical Audit Team.* Available from: www.hqip.org.uk/wp-content/uploads/2018/02/developing-clinical-audit-patient-panels.pdf

Hollnagel, E. (2022). Safety Synthesis – The Repository for Safety-II. Available form: www.safetysynthesis.com

Ikehara, H. T. (1999). Implications of gestalt theory and practice for the learning organisation. *The Learning Organisation*, 6(2), 63–69.

Khatri, N., Brown, G. D., & Hicks, L. L. (2009). From a blame culture to a just culture in health care. *Health Care Management Review*, 34(4), 312–322.

Kirkup, B. (2022). *Reading the signals: Maternity and neonatal services in East Kent – the Report of the Independent Investigation.* London: HM Stationary Office.

Marx, D. A. (2001). Patient safety and the 'just culture': A primer for health care executives. New York: Trustees of Columbia University.

Mersey Care NHS Foundation Trust. (2022). Restorative and Just Learning Culture. Available from: www.merseycare.nhs.uk/restorative-just-learning-culture

NHS England. (2015a). To huddle or not to huddle; Your essential guide. Available from: www.england.nhs.uk/signuptosafety/wp-content/uploads/sites/16/2015/11/huddles-essential-guide.pdf

NHS England. (2015b). *Serious Incident Framework: Supporting learning to prevent recurrence.* Available from: www.england.nhs.uk/patientsafety/wp-content/uploads/sites/32/2015/04/serious-incidnt-framwrk-upd2.pdf

NHS England (2020). *The patient safety incident response framework.* Available from: www.england.nhs.uk/patient-safety/incident-response-framework

NHS Improvement. (2018). *The future of NHS patient safety investigations.* London: NHS Improvement.

Peerally, M., Carr, S., Waring, J. & Dixon-Woods, M. (2017). The problem with root cause analysis. *BMJ Quality and Safety Journal*, 26(5), 417–422. Available from: https://qualitysafety.bmj.com/content/qhc/early/2016/06/23/bmjqs-2016-005511.full.pdf

Reason, J. (1997). *Managing the Risks of Organizational Accidents.* Ashgate Publishing.

Titcombe, J., & Montgomery, N. (2022). The NHS is still not learning from past mistakes in maternity. *Health Service Journal*, 5 April. Available from: www.hsj.co.uk/patient-safety/the-nhs-is-still-not-learning-from-past-mistakes-in-maternity/7032229.article

United States Agency for International Development. (2013). After-Action Review Guidance. Available from: https://usaidlearninglab.org/sites/default/files/resource/files/afteractionreviewguidancemarch2013.pdf

von Thaden, T., Hoppes, M., Li, Y., Johnson, N., & Schriver, A. (2006). The perception of just culture across disciplines in healthcare. *Proceedings of the Human Factors and Ergonomics Society Annual Meeting*, 50(10), 964–968.

Wang, C. L., & Ahmed, P. K. (2003). Organisational learning: A critical review. *The Learning Organization*, 10(1), 8–17.

# Glossary of terms

**Accountability**   being answerable/responsible/liable/culpable, and able to answer for and defend actions.

**Adverse childhood experiences (ACEs)**   stressful and distressing events and experiences that have occurred in childhood i.e. witnessing domestic violence, being subjected to childhood sexual/emotional abuse, neglect, violence, parental divorce/separation, abandonment, having a parent with a serious mental illness.

**After-action reviews (AARs)**   an approach to evaluation following an adverse event. AARs aim to avoid repetition of such events, and capture learning.

**Appreciative inquiry**   a strengths-based approach to organisational change, which emphasises a focus on the positives, rather than a more negative problem or deficit-based approach.

**Anti-task activities**   tasks engaged in by staff which are contrary to the primary task of an organisation. This may be because staff do not understand or agree with the primary task or may not understand what their own role or contribution should be, or because practice is influenced by **social defences** (see below).

**Asylum seeker**   adult, child, or young person whose request for sanctuary has yet to be processed by the government.

**Brexit**   the withdrawal of the United Kingdom from the European Union, following the 2016 Referendum.

**Burnout**   the result of poorly managed or unrecognised chronic workplace stress and dissatisfaction. It manifests with feelings of negativity and/or cynicism, lack of energy and enthusiasm, and feeling mentally 'removed/distant' – all in relation to work/role.

**Caldicott guardian**   a nominated person in a senior role in an organisation that needs to process individuals' health/social care personal data. The Caldicott guardian ensures that this personal data is used appropriately, ethically, and legally, and that the confidentiality of those who use their service in maintained. They may also provide expert guidance on matters that relate to information sharing and confidentiality.

**Care coordinator**   carries a case load of service users and is responsible for helping them to navigate the health/care system and to maintain an active role in their own care. Care coordinators work as part of a multi-disciplinary team, provide assessments in relation to mental health and risk, may provide or sign-post to specific interventions, and monitor in relation to medication.

**Child protection**   is focused on protecting children who have been identified as likely to or be suffering significant harm.

**Clinical audit**   uses established criteria to systematically assess whether day-to-day practice is congruent with organisational policy and best practice. Is used to ensure and support quality improvement in health care settings.

**Compassion fatigue**   a state of emotional, physical, and mental exhaustion as a result of the stress associated with exposure to repeated trauma.

**Compromised environment**   a country or region in which there are well-established perceptions of public sector corruption, extortion, abuse of authority for private gain, and any diplomatic, legal, or economic pressure being brought to bear on individuals by regional or other actors (including the host nation).

**Content analysis**   an evaluation/research tool, which analyses the words, concepts, and themes within text.

**Covid-19**   the global (pandemic) outbreak of the coronavirus, which was a highly contagious and severe respiratory disease.

**Critical consciousness**   an appreciation that we do not exist in isolation, and that knowledge and culture are ever changing.

**Debriefing**   a meeting following an event or piece of work, with those directly involved, to discuss what went well, or what went wrong, in an attempt to further organisational/team learning.

**Duty of candour**   the legal obligation in the UK for healthcare professionals to be open and honest with service users and their families/carers, when something has gone wrong with their care/treatment.

**Epistemic injustice**   the devaluing and/or dismissing of another's knowledge due to the prejudice of the hearer.

**Executive summary**   a short section of a report/document that summarises the longer document, so that the reader can quickly understand the large body of material contained, without having to read the entire report/document.

**Explicit bias**   our preferences for people, things, and groups, which we are consciously aware of (but may not share if we are aware reactions to them may be negative). Developed and shaped by our family and peer influences, media influences, and life experiences.

**Fishbone diagram**   a visual tool used as part of the root cause analysis methodology, to categorise the potential significant factors in relation to incident analysis.

**Fitness to practise (FtP)**   according to the Health and Care Professions Council (HCPC), someone is fit to practise if they have 'the skills, knowledge, character and health to practise their profession safely and effectively'. If practitioners fail to do this, they may become subject to a fitness to practise investigation, which may result in sanctions to their practice.

**Forced migration**   forced displacement from the place of origin, due to conflict, violence, or persecution.

**Francis Effect**   relates to the impact of the *Francis Report*.

**Francis Report**   an independent inquiry, chaired by Robert Francis, reported in February 2010, that failures in Mid Staffordshire in patient safety and care were caused by inadequate training of staff, staff cutbacks, and overemphasis on government targets.

**Freedom to Speak Up guardian**   support staff to articulate their concerns, especially when they are unable to do so using other systems/routes. They ensure that concerns raised are addressed and that the person raising the concern receives feedback on what actions have been taken.

**General Data Protection Regulation (GDPR)**   a European Union privacy and human rights law, which came into effect in 2018. It provides a legal framework for keeping individuals' personal information confidential, by requiring organisations to have robust systems, procedures, and training in relation to the processing and storage of personal data.

**General Medical Council (GMC)**   the public body that maintains the official register of medical practitioners in the United Kingdom, and sets standards for doctors' education, standards for patient care, and professional behaviour.

**Governance**   the actions and/or processes of overseeing or managing a department/organisation and maintaining quality.

**Health Care Professionals Council (HCPC)**   formerly the Health Professionals Council, a regulator of healthcare professionals from 15 health and care professions in the United Kingdom.

**Hostile environment**   a country or region that is subject to any war, insurrection, civil unrest, terrorism, or facing extreme levels of crime, banditry, lawlessness, or public disorder; typically, a complex or hazardous environment, characterised by its high risk and danger, often remote or difficult to access, with extreme climatic conditions or terrain and natural disasters, such as volcanoes, earthquakes, or tsunamis.

**Hot debrief**   a structured team-based discussion which may be initiated immediately following a significant event, whilst events are fresh in the mind of those involved.

**Hypermnesia**   vivid or abnormally comprehensive memory recall.

**Implicit bias**   the positive or negative preferences for individuals, groups, or things that have been shaped by our individual life experiences, family, and peers.

**Informants**   any individual involved in or affected by the serious incident, who may have relevant information to share that will inform the investigation.

**Just culture**   in healthcare, a just culture supports the fair treatment of staff, ensuring that they feel able to speak out when things have gone wrong, without fear of being blamed.

**Kolb's Experiential Learning Cycle**   according to Kolb, effective learning follows a four-stage cycle: concrete experience, reflective observation, abstract conceptualisation, and active experimentation.

**Lundy's Model of Participation**   a model of child participation, which has been adopted by organisations in the UK and abroad, to assist their understanding in relation to the participation of children and young people. The model is based on four key concepts:

- space – provision of a safe space where children and young people feel able to express themselves
- voice – provision of information and support, so that children and young people feel enabled to express their views
- audience – ensuring that the views expressed by children and young people are shared with relevant people
- influence — ensuring that the views of children and young people are taken seriously, and appropriate action taken.

**Mental Health Act (MHA) assessment**    an assessment as to whether an individual meets the criteria for compulsory detention under the Mental Health Act (1983), undertaken by an approved mental health professional (AMHP), a Section 12 approved doctor, and another registered medical practitioner.

**Nominal group technique**    a method for managing group discussions that structures the feedback and enables all voices to be heard. It can be used as a research methodology too.

**Nursing and Midwifery Council (NMC)**    the professional and regulatory body for nurses and midwives.

**Open systems model**    states that an organisation consists of economic, social, and political aspects, which impact on its functioning and success. Organisational processes, inputs/outputs, and goals enable the functioning of systems.

**Organisational culture**    the shared perspectives, expectations, approaches, and values of a team/department/service/organisation, which shape the practice of staff in that workplace.

**Paranoid schizophrenia**    a serious mental illness, in which the sufferer experiences a psychotic and delusional state which is marked by suspiciousness and fear of others.

**Patient Safety Incident Response Framework (PSIRF)**    issued by NHS England in 2022, with the aim of ensuring that organisations develop and maintain effective systems in relation to patient safety.

**Personality disorder**    a condition that affects how individuals relate to others, and can impact on thinking, feelings, and behaviour, often because of childhood trauma.

**Post-traumatic stress disorder**    the experience of anxiety related to previous traumatic events where the person believed that their life was in danger.

**Psychological safety**    the belief that views, ideas, and opinions can be expressed without fear of blame, punishment, judgement, or humiliation.

**Psychosis**    a mental health condition in which the sufferer experiences a range of symptoms (such as hallucinations and delusions) which mean they may not be able to differentiate between what is real and what is not, but lack the insight to appreciate this.

**Rapid review**    conducted as an alternative to a more in-depth approach when a review needs to be completed quickly.

**Reciprocity** sometimes also referred to as 'mutuality', where people work for the benefit of each other.

**Refugee** adult, child, or young person whose application for asylum has been accepted by the UK government as meeting the definition of refugee in the Refugee Convention, resulting in refugee status documentation. In the UK, refugees are usually granted five years leave to remain as a refugee, after which they need to apply for further leave.

**Restorative Just Culture** a culture of fairness and transparency which enables learning. It aims to facilitate openness and a forum that invites 'speaking up' without fear of blame or retribution, to learn from and prevent mistakes reoccurring.

**Root cause analysis (RCA)** a structured approach to solving problems by identifying the root causes of the problem, assuming that it is better to treat the underlying issue than treat the symptoms.

**Safeguarding** a process which protects a person's health, wellbeing, and rights from abuse, harm, or neglect.

**Safety huddle** a group of people, usually standing (rather than seated), that meet to discuss an issue of safety or risk to inform and create swift, collaborative actions.

**Safety-I approach** an approach to patient safety investigations in which there is a focus on what has gone wrong.

**Safety-II approach** an approach to patient safety investigations in which there is a focus on what has been done well, as this also enables consideration and understanding of what may have gone wrong.

**Schizophrenia** a psychotic illness (see above).

**Second victims** people who have been involved in an unanticipated, adverse incident such as a patient safety incident or adverse event, or a medical error, and then feel traumatised.

**Self-awareness** insight into ourselves and our actions. Sometimes described as knowing ourselves.

**Semi-permissive environments** a specific environment in which the local-national or international security forces operating within can expect to experience variable degrees of obstruction, interference, and resistance, alongside challenges to their authority. The local security situation will likely be volatile and unstable, with restrictions placed on the local movement and international travel of civilians and foreign nationals created by an inability of the host nation to fully impose law and order.

**Significant incident learning process** a whole systems approach to learning from events, in which the perspectives and experiences of staff involved in adverse events, and organisational systems, are considered and evaluated.

**Social defences** happens when employees experience stress/anxiety and unconsciously collude to protect themselves from this by engaging in activities/tasks unrelated to the primary function/task of that workplace.

**Stereotypes** our automatic associations in relation to people, groups, and things, which can be positive or negative.

**Stigma**    the social consequences of negative attributions.

**Structured judgement review**    Royal College of Physicians methodology, intended for use in adult in-patient environments, in which clinicians use explicit standards to evaluate the quality of healthcare.

**Terms of reference**    define the scope, purpose, and approach taken during an investigation

**Thematic analysis**    a systematic and structured scrutiny of a passage of text (e.g. a narrative or a transcription) which identifies recurring issues of significance.

**Transactional positioning**    relates to perceived fairness in employment settings, and the consequences of perceived unfairness/fairness on behaviour.

**Unaccompanied asylum-seeking child (UASC)**    young people who have journeyed to the UK unaccompanied by a parent or legal guardian. They are automatically a looked after child, under the care of the local authority. They have full entitlement to free NHS care and other public services. NHS charging regulations do not apply to them.

**Unconscious bias**    see 'implicit bias'.

**Undocumented migrant**    a term often used to refer to people who do not have any formal immigration status/leave to remain. People without leave to remain also do not have recourse to public funds.

**Welsh Model**    the Child Practice Review Framework developed in Wales in 2015, in which practitioners are involved in evaluating issues as a way of ensuring more meaningful insights, and more relevant, achievable, and proportionate recommendations.

**World Health Organization (WHO)**    founded in 1948, the United Nations agency that connects nations, partners, and people to promote health, keep the world safe, and serve the vulnerable.

# Index

Note: Page numbers in *italic* indicate a figure, **bold** a table.

Printed in the United States
by Baker & Taylor Publisher Services